MAXIMIZING YOUR HEALTH AND VITALITY

Juicing has come of age—the connection between good health and good nutrition has been proven beyond a doubt. And now, with the help of this invaluable book, you can whip up your own delicious fresh fruit and vegetable juices. Find out:

- all about "anutrients" and how they can prevent disease
- which are the best juices for healthy babies, toddlers, and children—how to prevent food allergies, ear infections, and more
- how to deliver the necessary nutrients to adolescents and young adults
- all about juicing for successful conception, pregnancy, and lactation
- how to relieve menopausal symptoms naturally through nutrition
- the disease-prevention diet for mature adults

From *A*pple to *W*atermelon, from *A*sparagus to *T*urnip greens, here is your guide to vibrant health and exuberant vitality at every age—*the natural way!*

MAUREEN B. KEANE is a licensed nutritionist, a member of the Society for Nutrition Education, and a part-time instructor at Bastyr College. She writes a monthly column on children's nutrition for *Choices,* a magazine for the owners of juice extractors. She lives in Seattle with her husband and son.

Juicing

For Good Health

MAUREEN B. KEANE

POCKET BOOKS

New York   London   Toronto   Sydney   Tokyo   Singapore

This book is intended to supplement, not replace, the advice of a trained health professional. If you know or suspect that you have a health problem, you should consult your doctor.

An *Original* Publication of POCKET BOOKS

 POCKET BOOKS, a division of Simon & Schuster Inc.
1230 Avenue of the Americas, New York, NY 10020

CONTENTS

CONTENTS

Part III: Juicing Through the Life Cycle

FOREWORD

Juicing has become one of today's hottest fads. I say that hesitantly because although it is great to see so many people drinking fresh fruit and vegetable juices, I fear it is for the wrong reasons. Americans love quick fixes. We see an energetic juice machine salesman on television and in the back of our minds we expect to look and feel like him after only a few days or weeks of juicing. When we don't shed our infirmities after a few days and a few glasses, we give up. Please don't. A glass of juice is not a quick fix or a shortcut to health. Nutrition does not work like that. Nutrition exerts a persistent nudging action that gently guides your body to health. In order for juicing to give you more energy and to help you live longer, it must be accompanied by the dietary changes recommended in each chapter. Remember, juicing is only one part of a healthy lifestyle that must also include exercise. Don't let it become a fad for you. Keep your juicer on the kitchen counter and let it give you years of enjoyment and health. It can truly become one of your best investments.

PART

— I —

Diet and Aging

CHAPTER ONE

An Introduction to Juicing

According to the *Oxford English Dictionary*, the word *chemical* comes from the Greek word *chemia*, which means "plant juice." For centuries, plant juices and extracts have been used for their healing and medicinal effects. Today, with modern methods of creating drugs and chemicals that have never before existed, we have forgotten about the original natural drugs nature has given us—fruits and vegetables.

WHAT IS JUICE?

In order to understand what juice is, we must first understand a little about the anatomy of a plant. Plant tissue, of course, varies according to which part of the plant the tissue is taken from. The composition of the roots of a plant is different from the composition of its leaves. However, most plant cells have the same fundamental structure.

PLANT CELLS

Plant cells are basically similar to animal cells. They consist of a nucleus that contains the genetic material of the plant and is surrounded by cytoplasm, which is composed of water, proteins, lipids, and other factors needed for growth and development. Membrane-enclosed storage sacs called vacuoles fill part of the cytoplasm. Vacuoles contain starch, sugar, proteins, wastes, and water-soluble pigments. Also inside the cytoplasm are structures unique to plants—the plastids. These structures can contain chlorophyll (chloroplasts), fat-soluble pigments (chromoplasts), or stored starch, protein, or lipid (leukoplasts). Surrounding the cytoplasm and its structures is the cell membrane, which in turn is surrounded by the cell wall, another feature unique to plants. The cell wall provides structure and rigidity to the plant. The spaces between cells can contain air (some apples contain as much as 25 percent air), and substances called pectins. Pectin is gel-like soluble fiber that acts as intercellular cement. The individual characteristics of plants are determined by these structures. The color of the plant is determined by the number and type of pigments in the chromoplasts, chloroplasts, and vacuoles, its texture is determined by the size of the cell wall, and its nutritive value and taste are determined by the contents of the vacuoles.

When a vegetable such as a carrot is put into a juice extractor, the cell walls are split open and the cytoplasm and other liquid components are separated from the cell walls and other fibrous parts of the plant. The liquid portion, or juice, contains the contents of the plastids and vacuoles, any vitamins, minerals, and flavor components that were present in the cytoplasm, and some of the pectins. The solid portions of the plant or pulp contain the cellulose, lignin, and the remaining pectins found in the cell walls. Juices are not a whole food, because they lack fiber, but they are a wholesome food, because they contain so many raw, unprocessed food components. The National Cancer Institute has recommended that Americans eat a minimum of five servings of fruits and vegetables each day. Many Americans find this a difficult level to achieve. Fruit and vegetable juices fresh from your juicer are an easy way to provide additional nutrition to your diet. They should not be viewed as a substitute for raw fruits and vegetables, but as an easy-to-make, delicious-to-drink supplement. But before you can begin to enjoy the benefits of juices, you must have a juicer.

HOW TO CHOOSE A JUICER

Juicers seem to be everywhere these days. Late-night television is full of "infomercials," half-hour commercials that urge you to buy a juice machine by calling their toll-free number. Health food stores also sell well-promoted, but expensive, machines. On the other hand, department and discount stores sell some models whose prices sometimes seem too good to be true. What's a person to do? Relax. Follow these guidelines and buying tips and you will be sure that it will be your veggies, not your wallet, that are getting juiced.

TYPES OF JUICERS

Juicers come in three basic types. The first is the **masticating juicer.** This type of machine grinds the plant into a soft mush and then squeezes the juice out through a screen. The Champion® Juicer is an example of this type.

The second type is the **centrifugal juicer.** Blades at the bottom of a spinning stainless-steel basket help to chew up the plant. The juice is then propelled through the screen on the sides of the basket and out the spout. The pulp is retained within the basket and must be removed after each batch of juice is made. An example of this is the Acme® juicer.

The **centrifugal juicer with pulp ejector** is the third type. This machine is basically the same as the centrifugal juicer, except that the pulp is ejected from the basket and collected in a pulp container. This type of machine does not need to be cleaned after each use. An example of this type is the Juiceman® Juicer.

I have been asked by many people what kind of juicer I recommend. My answer is always the same. The best juicer for you is a juicer that you will use consistently. It doesn't matter how fancy a machine it is, or how efficiently it extracts juice, or how cheap it is. If a juicer does not fit your lifestyle, you will eventually grow tired of using it, and it will be retired to the appliance graveyard.

POINTS TO REMEMBER WHEN BUYING A JUICER

- Remember that you are not purchasing health or longevity, you are buying a household appliance. Never buy a machine unless you have personally inspected the brand and model. I recommend that you do not buy a juicer after only seeing a television demonstration. Some of the brands advertised on television are excellent machines, but some of them are also overpriced junk. Unfortunately, the magic of TV makes some of the cheaper models appear to do a better job than they are able.

• Ask your friends who have juicers to describe the good and bad points of their machines. Which features do they think are worth the extra money? Would they purchase that machine again? Some extra features on juicing machines may lose their appeal after a while, and you may wish you had bought a simpler model.

• Compare prices and models in at least three stores. Start at a health food store. Health food stores tend to carry the more expensive machines, but their salespeople are well-informed. Become familiar with the features of the most expensive machines so that you will recognize them on less-expensive models. Listen and look, but don't buy yet. The next stop is the department store. Here you will find juicers made by the manufactures of other kitchen appliances. Evaluate the models according to the guidelines below, but don't buy yet. Lastly, try a discount warehouse. These stores often carry the machines shown on television as well as department store brands at greatly reduced prices. This is a good opportunity to examine some of the infomercial machines.

TEN GUIDELINES FOR EVALUATING A JUICER

When you go into a store to evaluate juicers keep these guidelines in mind:

1. Pick up the machine. How heavy is it? Is it light and flimsy or heavy and sturdy? The heavier machines are often the most durable. On the other hand, machines that are too heavy will be difficult for some individuals to lift. If you have arthritis, or suffer from a loss of muscle strength, make sure you choose a juicer that is manageable for you.

2. Look at the quality of the plastic on the machine. Is it strong and of good quality, or is it cheap and thin? A juicer that is cheap on the outside is not likely to be of high quality on the inside.

3. Take the juicer apart and put it back together again. How easy is it to assemble and disassemble? Are there too many parts? How easy will it be to clean? If you have arthritis or another chronic illness that reduces hand strength, this is a very important point to evaluate.

4. How large is the pulp container? A small receptacle means you will have to empty the container more often. How easy will it be to clean? Sharp corners may be difficult to pry pulp out of.

5. How large is the feeder tube? The smaller the tube, the more cutting and chopping you will have to do to fit the produce through.

6. How much space does the juicer occupy? Since your juice machine will be used every day, it should not be put away, but installed in a permanent spot on your kitchen counter. Choose a juicer that will fit your counter space.

7. Read the booklet that accompanies the machine. How do they recommend that you prepare the fruits and vegetables? Is the motor strong enough to handle skins and rinds, or must everything be peeled? Again, the more preparation you have to do, the less likely you will be to use your juicer.

8. Does the machine come with a warranty? What kind of service can you expect if the machine breaks?

If the juicer does not meet your expectations, will the store you buy it from allow you to return it?

9. As soon as you have bought your juicer, try juicing carrots and apples immediately. If the motor jams, or if the pulp is not ejected properly and it plugs up the machine, return the juicer to the store immediately and choose another model.

10. Does the style of the juicer match the style of your life? If you have no time for cleaning and even less time for eating, do not choose a juicer with extra attachments that may be difficult to clean. Consider purchasing a centrifugal juicer with a pulp ejector. If you have arthritis and have difficulty preparing fruits and vegetables for juicing, consider investing in a juicer with a powerful motor and large intake tube that will require a minimum of peeling and chopping. Masticating juicers can also make great "ice cream" from frozen fruits, as well as grind nuts and seeds. If you have ice cream–addicted kids, this machine can become a family favorite.

If at all possible, borrow a machine before you buy one. This is particularly advantageous if you are leaning towards higher-priced models. After you have evaluated the machines, pick the top three models that fit your lifestyle and pocketbook. Call around to various stores to find the lowest price on these models, and then purchase one you can afford. If you get it home and it does not live up to your expectations, return it to the store and select a model that will work.

Again, it is important to remember that a cheap juicer is not a bargain if it is too difficult to use. In the end, you will only use a juicer that is easy to clean and easy to prepare produce for.

CHAPTER TWO

Aging

Is the fountain of youth stashed away in your kitchen cupboard? Could your juicer be the source of the famed elixir that Ponce de Leon searched for in vain? Unfortunately, a glass or two of fresh juice each day cannot turn back the clock and transform you into a strapping youth. However, a whole foods diet, with plenty of fruits and vegetables supplemented by fresh juices, can make a difference in the length and quality of your life. To understand how good nutrition and consistent juicing can accomplish this, we must first understand how and why the body ages, what factors affect the aging process, and how foods can modify these factors.

WHAT IS AGING?

Life expectancy and longevity are terms we hear a lot of these days. They refer to the average number of years an *individual* can expect to live. Life span, on the other hand, refers to the maximum number of years that a *species* can expect to live. Life expectancy at the turn of the century was 47 years. Infectious diseases such as smallpox, tuberculosis, diphtheria, tetanus, and rheumatic fever were the major killers. Today, the average American lives for 75 years, and that number is constantly rising. The major killer diseases are now degenerative diseases such as coronary heart disease, cancer, and diabetes. Slowly but surely, our life expectancy is approaching our life span. The oldest living human died at the age of 120, and many researchers believe that for as yet unknown reasons, this is the longest that the human body can survive.

Many individuals feel that the best time of their lives is middle age, when they have achieved the physical and mental maturity to accomplish the goals they have set for themselves. Yet for many people this period is cut short by death or disability due to disease. Why do chronic diseases cut short our life expectancy? Why can't we live forever if we avoid chronic disease? Nobody knows for certain why the body ages, although it is the subject of much discussion and research.

These are some of the most promising and exciting theories on the process of aging:

PROGRAMMED AGING

The programmed aging theory suggests that aging is somehow programmed into our genetic code much as instructions are programmed into a computer. It views aging as a continuation of the same kind of genetic program that supervised the development of our bodies from egg to embryo to mature individual.

It sees aging and death as the result of an orderly series of biological events, similar to the mechanism that kills salmon after spawning.

Supporters of this theory point out that: identical twins have a greater similarity between the length of their lives than do fraternal twins; long-lived individuals are usually found in families with long-lived ancestors; and the life span of cells grown in tissue cultures is directly related to the age and life span of the cell donor. And although evidence suggests that longevity is related to heredity, it does not mean that the physical changes that accompany aging are under genetic control.

ERROR-CATASTROPHE THEORY

The error-catastrophe or "wear and tear" theory implies that aging is the result of an accumulation of a lifetime of exposure to harmful environmental influences. This exposure eventually threatens a cell's ability to survive. Proponents of this theory argue that random errors in the manufacture of protein might accumulate and eventually damage cells. A major argument against this theory is that cells have the ability to "proofread" proteins and break down those that have been altered. Since this ability declines with age, it may be that the accumulation of altered proteins is the result of lower rates of degradation of altered proteins, not higher rates of error in protein manufacture.

DNA DAMAGE AND REPAIR THEORY

The genetic material of a cell is vulnerable to damage from many sources. In order to prevent this damage from interfering with cell duplication, most organisms have evolved DNA repair mechanisms. The more effective a cell is at preventing, recognizing, and repairing DNA damage, the slower the aging process becomes. Evidence to support this theory has been difficult to obtain, because it was impossible to examine and measure the DNA repair system. Only recently have the proper molecular tools for the examination of this theory been developed. It may be that the lack of DNA repair mechanisms is responsible for the aging of some types of tissues, but not all.

FREE RADICAL THEORY

A free radical is a molecule that has a single unpaired electron in its outer orbit. Electrons have a compulsion to travel in pairs, and molecules that lack an electron will go to almost any length to acquire a new partner. They react with proteins, genetic material, and the lipid (fat) part of cell membranes. Once the free radical has acquired its new partner, it is no longer reactive. However, the molecule that had its electron stolen now becomes a free radical and in turn steals electrons from other molecules. This creates a chain reaction that progressively causes more and more damage.

Lipid peroxidation is one well-studied mechanism of free radical injury to cells. It occurs when free radicals attack the unsaturated fatty acids that are a part of the cell membranes and produce organic acid-free radicals. These free radicals quickly react with oxygen to form peroxides. Peroxides then act as free radicals themselves, resulting in a further loss of unsaturated fatty acids and extensive damage to the cell membrane. Because free radicals are so plentiful in the environment, the body has developed two mechanisms to protect itself from them. These are the antioxidant nutrients and the antioxidant enzymes.

1. Antioxidants are molecules that prevent oxidation, or reactions with oxygen. Some antioxidants are made by the body (cysteine and glutathione) and some are supplied by the diet (vitamins C and E). Antioxidants are like soldiers on a search-and-destroy mission. They seek out free radicals (scavenge) and react with them to inactivate (quench) them, breaking the chain reaction of damage.

2. Enzymes produced by the body also quench free radicals. These include superoxide dismutase, catalase, and glutathione peroxidase.

This theory proposes that the aging process is the sum of injurious free radical reactions going on continuously throughout the cells and tissues. According to this theory, much depends on defense mechanisms such as vitamin E and selenium-containing glutathione peroxidase and other antioxidants for the prevention or slowing of cellular aging. Researchers who support this theory point to studies that show that the life expectancy of lab animals is increased by antioxidants. Critics, however, point out that life span is not. Free radicals may cause specific chronic diseases that in turn contribute to aging, but they are not directly responsible for shortening your life.

MULTIFACTORIAL THEORY

The aging of an organism occurs on many different levels: molecular, cellular, and of the organs themselves. Because of the complexity involved, it is unlikely that one single mechanism could be responsible for all of these changes. What we perceive as aging is probably the sum of a number of different factors, mechanisms, and genes.

Since science does not yet know the cause of aging and has yet to find a way to expand the human life span, let us concentrate on what we can do to increase our life expectancy and our health expectancy.

A NEW VIEW OF AGING

As we approach the latter half of life expectancy, our bodily functions begin to slow down. We shake our heads sadly at our inability to duplicate the frantic pace of our youth and blame all our problems on "aging." If longevity is your goal, you must develop a new outlook on aging. Aging is not a thief who sneaks up on you and suddenly steals your "youth." Aging is a process that includes being young. It is a journey that begins at conception and winds through all the cycles of life, ending only at the final heartbeat. It is a journey filled with change and evolution, each individual cycle having its ups and downs, good times and bad times. In order to successfully negotiate our pilgrimage through the life cycles, we must learn to adapt our ways of living and our ways of eating to accommodate the cycle we are in. As teenagers, we must increase our energy intake to accommodate the huge increases in growth rate. In middle age, we must decrease our energy intake to compensate for the decreased rate of growth. As seniors we must increase nutrients to compensate for decreased absorption. This process of adaptation and accommodation will help us increase our health expectancy as well as our life expectancy.

HEALTH EXPECTANCY

Life expectancy is the number of years that one can expect to live. Health expectancy is the number of years that one can expect to live and be healthy and active, without disabilities or chronic diseases. A long life without health is pointless. Of what use is it to expand the number of years we live if those years cannot be happy and productive? Although it is a fact of life that we will age, it is also a fact that people can age at different rates. Health expectancy can be increased by following a healthy diet and lifestyle. Here are some of the factors that affect your chances of living a longer and more productive life:

1. *Genetics.* How long you live and how fast you age is in some part genetic. Many researchers believe that the best way to ensure a long life is to choose your parents well. Some forms of cancer are inherited, along with some forms of heart disease. They are, however, the exception rather than the rule. It is usually a tendency to develop a disease that is inherited, not the disease itself. These tendencies must be activated by certain environmental conditions before they are expressed. For example, the tendency to develop type II diabetes can be inherited. Individuals with a family history of diabetes can reduce the amount of calories they consume and increase the fiber and nutrient content of their diets, thereby preventing the disease from ever developing. Some people inherit a sensitivity to salt, which causes their blood pressure to rise when too much salt is consumed. By reducing salt intake these individuals can prevent the development of hypertension. If you know certain diseases "run" in your family, begin a prevention program now. A healthy diet and lifestyle

can serve only as damage control once the disease has developed.

2. *Lifestyle.* Many individuals choose a lifestyle that is more of a "deathstyle." Poor lifestyle choices include the use of tobacco, overuse of alcohol, recreational drug use, and skin tanning. All of these activities can contribute to premature aging, chronic disease, and eventually, death.

3. *Diet.* Fruits and vegetables, along with other plant foods, contain a myriad of chemicals. Some of the chemicals are the antioxidant nutrients beta-carotene, vitamin C, vitamin E, and the mineral selenium. These antioxidants help to prevent free radical damage. Free radicals may not be the sole cause of aging, but they are definitely a major factor in cellular injury. Mounting evidence suggests that they can prevent or at least delay many of the diseases associated with aging, including cancer, cataracts, diabetes, heart disease, suppressed immune function, Parkinson's disease, and periodontal disease.

Other substances have been dubbed "anutrients." These substances include: plant pigments such as the carotenoids (yellow and red), chlorophyll (green), anthocyanins (reddish), proanthocyanidins ("colorless"), flavonoids (yellow), and tannins (colorless, yellow, and brown); antiviral, antifungal, and antibacterial compounds that protect plants from microbes in the environment; and pungent odors and flavors that plants use to repel would-be consumers. Many researchers speculate that man has developed the ability to adopt and utilize the protective capacity of these substances when they are eaten. These substances play many roles in the human body, ranging from antioxidants and blood thinners to cancer-blocking and suppressive agents to anti-inflammatory agents.

Research has shown that a high consumption of fruits and vegetables lowers the risk of developing cancer. The Western culture consumes a diet with a certain set of cancer-causing and -promoting agents. The Oriental culture consumes a diet with a different set of cancer-causing and -promoting agents. Yet in all cases the risk of developing cancer is reduced by a regular intake of fruits and vegetables. No matter what the carcinogens and promoters are, no matter where the culture is located, the results are always the same. At the beginning of this century we worried about nutrient deficiencies. Deficiency diseases such as pellagra (niacin) were not uncommon. Today there is a shift toward degenerative diseases such as cancer and heart disease. These diseases can be prevented to a large extent by eating fruits and vegetables. Despite that knowledge, we still do not eat enough fruits and vegetables. According to a government telephone survey, on any given day a large portion of the American public eats no vegetables or fruit. We are no longer suffering from vitamin deficiencies; our real problem is now vegetable deficiencies.

HOW TO CURE YOUR VEGETABLE DEFICIENCY

We are creatures of habit, and many of us have never gotten the vegetable habit. It is not as difficult as it sounds. Every morning have a whole-grain cereal with fresh fruit sliced on top (1 serving). Lunch should be accompanied by a salad with a cup of raw vegetables (1 serving), and bring a whole piece of fruit to work for an afternoon snack (1 serving). Include two different vegetables (other than potatoes) with dinner (2 servings). That adds up to the five servings that the National Academy of Sciences recommends. Additional insurance is provided by adding juices to your diet. In the morning have a glass of fresh citrus juice, and in the evening have a large glass of vegetable juice. Every morning and every evening, every day. Make it a habit and kick your vegetable deficiency.

PART
── II ──
Juicing for Prevention

CHAPTER THREE

Coronary Heart Disease

Coronary heart disease, or CHD, is the number one killer of Americans today. It is by far the leading cause of death in men over 35 and although we tend to think of heart disease as a male problem, it kills men and women equally over 45. About five million Americans have been diagnosed with CHD and it has been estimated that a majority of adult Americans have mild undiagnosed cases. Since many of the risk factors for CHD are influenced by the foods we eat, this disease can be prevented in many people by proper diet.

WHAT IS CORONARY HEART DISEASE?

When the heart beats, it pumps blood to two sets of arteries: the arteries that supply the heart (coronary arteries) and the arteries that supply the body. When the coronary arteries are not able to deliver a sufficient amount of blood to the heart muscle, the result is CHD. This lack of oxygen to the muscle cells can produce chest pain (angina pectoris) and difficulty in breathing (dyspnea). If the arteries become totally blocked, all blood is cut off to a part of the heart, resulting in the death of those muscle cells. This is called a myocardial infarction (MI) or heart attack.

WHAT CAUSES CHD?

CHD is caused by a narrowing of the coronary arteries by atherosclerosis. Atherosclerosis is the process by which fibrous lesions or *plaques* are formed in the innermost lining of the arteries. It is thought that the lining of the artery is somehow injured and that this injury allows cholesterol and lipid to be deposited in the muscle in the artery lining. Over time these deposits or plaques become covered by a cap of smooth muscle and fibrous tissue that then begins to protrude into the center of the artery. As these plaques grow, they reduce the flow of blood through the artery. This progressive narrowing can totally close off an artery blocking blood flow or the narrowed opening can be blocked by a blood clot.

HOW DIET CAN HELP
TO PREVENT CHD

Prevention of heart disease by diet focuses on several different areas.

1. Plaque formation in the arteries may be prevented by protecting the vulnerable lining of the artery from free radical damage. If you have had a blood cholesterol test done recently, you are probably

familiar with the term "low density lipoproteins" or LDL. LDL is commonly referred to as the "bad" cholesterol. The LDL molecule can become damaged by free radicals forming oxidized LDL, a very toxic molecule that may damage the muscle cells lining the arteries. This can cause new plaques to form or old plaques to become larger from new deposits of cholesterol. The transformation from LDL to oxidized LDL can be prevented by two types of compounds: antioxidant nutrients and antioxidant enzymes. Antioxidant nutrients, vitamins C and E and the carotenoids, protect lipid membranes from free radical attack. Both types of antioxidants work by protecting the lipid membrane from free radical attack. Antioxidant nutrients include: vitamin C, vitamin E, and beta-carotene. Antioxidant enzymes include: glutathione peroxidase (which contains selenium) and superoxide dismutase (which requires copper, zinc, and manganese).

2. Some minerals reduce the size of plaques. The mechanism involved is unknown. Examples are: magnesium, chromium, and copper.

3. Some nutrients prevent the overgrowth of smooth muscle cells that are part of plaque formation. Vitamin E is an example of this.

4. The amount of cholesterol circulating in the blood can be reduced by certain nutrients. The omega-3 fatty acids found in certain fish can reduce cholesterol levels. The soluble fiber found in carrots, apples, and oats binds with cholesterol in the intestine and prevents its reabsorption. Niacin, a B vitamin, when taken in therapeutic doses is very effective in lowering cholesterol levels in the blood. This treatment, however, must be supervised by a physician because of the possibility of liver damage. Plant sterols such as B-sitosterol and brassicasterol can block the intestine from absorbing dietary cholesterol.

5. Some nutrients raise HDL (high density lipoproteins, called "good" cholesterol) levels. Examples of this are vitamin C and beta-carotene.

6. Some nutrients are able to prevent the formation of blood clots. Garlic contains four compounds that inhibit blood clotting, the most potent being ajoene. Unidentified compounds in onions, cantaloupe, and ginger root also reduce clot formation.

DIETARY CHANGES
TO PREVENT HEART DISEASE

1. Reduce the total amount of saturated fat in your diet. A diet high in the saturated fat that comes from animals is linked to high cholesterol levels. Sources of saturated fat include all red meat, poultry, and whole milk products such as cheese, butter, ice cream and yogurt. Replace these foods with their nonfat versions.

2. Eat more soy foods. Nutrients in soybeans aid in lowering cholesterol levels in some people. Soy products include: soybeans, tofu, tempeh, and fortified soymilk.

3. Replace polyunsaturated fats (PUFAs) with monounsaturated fats (MUFAs). Monounsaturates lower the risk of CHD without increasing the risk for cancer. Oils that contain high amounts of MUFAs include: olive oil, canola oil, and high oleic safflower oil.

4. Eat large amounts of onions, garlic, cantaloupe, and ginger. These foods will help to prevent blood clots.

5. Eat foods high in soluble fiber. Soluble fiber acts as a sponge in the intestine, soaking up cholesterol and preventing the body from reabsorbing and recycling it. **Foods that contain soluble fiber include: fruits, vegetables, physillium seed, and oats.**

6. Eat more cold water fish such as salmon, mackerel, herring, whitefish, lake trout, and halibut. The omega-3 fatty acids in these fish may help to lower cholesterol levels, as well as reduce the risk of blood clotting. Several studies have found that these fish oils have a protective effect on the reoccurrence of coronary restenosis after angioplasty. Remember that fish oil supplements work best when you take them with fish.

7. Eat foods rich in the antioxidant nutrients. These foods will help to protect the arteries in your heart from free radical damage. Sweet peppers, vegetables in the cabbage family, and fruits in the citrus family are excellent sources of vitamin C. Sunflower seeds, almonds, olive oil, and wheat germ are good sources of vitamin E. Orange-fleshed fruits such as papaya and cantaloupe, orange-colored vegetables such as carrots and sweet potatoes, and green leafy vegetables such as spinach and kale are all excellent sources of beta-carotene and the other carotenoids. Wheat germ and whole grains, shellfish such as scallops and shrimp, Brazil nuts and orange juice are good sources of selenium.

8. Sprinkle sliced almonds, walnuts, and sunflower seeds on your veggies and salads. Almonds are rich in fiber, monounsaturated fats, copper and magnesium. Walnuts are high in omega-3 fatty acids and copper. Sunflower seeds are rich in vitamin E and magnesium.

JUICES TO PREVENT HEART DISEASE

Apple: source of chromium and pectin

Asparagus: source of vitamin E and beta-carotene
Cantaloupe: source of beta-carotene and adenosine (a natural blood thinner)
Carrot: source of carotenoids, copper, and selenium
Garlic: source of ajoene and copper
Ginger: source of zinc, and blood thinning compound
Green peppers: source of vitamin C and chromium
Kale: source of carotenoids, vitamin C, calcium, and magnesium
Orange: source of vitamin C and selenium
Spinach: source of vitamin E, carotenes, and chromium

JUICE RECIPES

High-C Veggie

This drink is rich in vitamin C and chromium.

1 green pepper
1 small handful spinach
2 carrots, tops removed

Juice ingredients. Garnish with a slice of pepper.

Triple Orange Carotene Cooler

This drink is loaded with beta-carotene and selenium.

¼ cantaloupe
1 orange, peeled
1 carrot, top removed

Prepare cantaloupe according to the instructions of your juicer. Juice all ingredients and serve immediately.

Heart Happy Veggie Drink

This drink contains blood-thinning compounds as well as all the antioxidants.

2 garlic cloves, peeled
3 carrots, tops removed
1 kale leaf
2 spears asparagus

Juice ingredients and drink immediately.

Heart Happy Fruit Drink

A sweeter version with blood thinners and antioxidant nutrients.

¼ cantaloupe
½-inch slice ginger root
½ cup strawberries
1 orange, peeled

Prepare cantaloupe according to the directions of your juicer. Remove green caps from strawberries and juice ingredients. Garnish with an orange slice.

Green E Juice

This juice is rich in vitamin E as well as chromium.

1 handful spinach
2 asparagus spears
1 green pepper
1 carrot, top removed

Juice ingredients. Garnish with a thin asparagus spear and serve immediately.

Fruity Trace Mineral Drink

This drink contains selenium, chromium, copper, and zinc.

2 oranges, peeled
1 apple, cored
½- to 1-inch slice ginger root
crushed ice

Juice ingredients and pour over ice. Garnish with an orange slice.

Pink Power Veggie Drink

Loaded with vitamin C, beta-carotene, and blood thinners, this drink will keep your heart in the pink.

1 sweet red pepper
¼ small onion
3 carrots, tops removed

Juice ingredients and garnish with a carrot curl and a slice of red pepper.

Pink Power Fruit Drink

This drink is loaded with vitamin C, beta-carotene, and blood thinners.

1 guava
½ mango
¾-inch slice ginger root
crushed ice

Juice ingredients, pour over ice, and serve immediately.

Triple Leaf Juice

This juice is high in beta-carotene, calcium, and vitamin C.

1 collard leaf
1 kale leaf
2 lettuce leaves
1 cucumber

If cucumber is waxed or not organic, remove peel. Juice ingredients and garnish with an asparagus spear.

CHAPTER FOUR

Cancer

Cancer is the second leading cause of death in the United States. About one in three people now living will develop cancer and one in five will die from it. Depressing statistics until you realize that 80 or maybe even 90 percent of all cancers may be caused by the environment and up to 60 percent may be diet related. This means that you can prevent many cancers by avoiding substances that are known to cause cancer. However, some cancer-causing substances are hidden in the environment. For help in protecting yourselves from these hidden threats you must turn to the plant kingdom. Many fruits and vegetables contain protective agents that, when eaten, will guard your body against the sneak attacks of cancer-causing substances.

WHAT IS CANCER?

In healthy tissue, cell division is an orderly process in which cells are produced for replacement or growth. Cancer occurs when these cells begin to reproduce, without need, at an uncontrollable rate and eventually spread to other areas of the body. Although we usually think of cancer as one disease, it is actually a very large group of very different diseases. There are as many different cancers as there are tissues of the body. Although cancer can occur anywhere in the body, cancers of the lung, colon-rectum, and breast are the most common.

WHAT CAUSES CANCER?

Cancer is caused by *carcinogens* or cancer-causing substances. Carcinogens can be viruses, chemicals, or radiant energy. Very few cancers are inherited. Most are caused by carcinogens in the environment or by an interaction of carcinogens with a genetic inclination. This means that most cancers are preventable. A cell becomes cancerous in two stages. The first stage is called *initiation*, which is produced by exposing cells to a cancer-causing agent or initiator. This exposure somehow changes the cell, making it more likely to become cancerous. The effect of an initiator is permanent, nothing can be done to reverse it. The second stage is *promotion*. A promoter causes an initiated cell to develop into a tumor but will not cause tumor development by itself. Fortunately the effects of a promoter on the cell are reversible. In order for a cancer to form, both initiation and promotion must take place.

HOW DIET CAN HELP
TO PREVENT CANCER

Carcinogens can be viruses, the by-products of intestinal bacteria, chemicals made by industry, chemicals added to foods, natural toxins, or radiation from the sun. The list of potential carcinogens is so enormous it is impossible to avoid all of them and still lead a productive and fulfilling life. That is why a healthy diet is so important. Agents present in food can actually prevent initiation and promotion of cancers. Some of the mechanisms are discussed below.

1. Some nutrients in foods prevent the formation of cancer-causing compounds from precursor compounds. Vitamin C and vitamin E have this type of action. For example, vitamin C prevents the nitrites present in food from forming cancer-causing nitrosamines in the stomach.

2. Some nutrients act as "blocking agents." These agents prevent cancer-causing substances from reaching or reacting with tissues by creating a barrier between the carcinogen and its target. Examples of blocking agents include: aromatic isothiocyanates, glucobrassicin, and indoles that are found in the cabbage family (Brussels sprouts, cabbage, kale, and broccoli); the organosulfur compounds found in the members of the Allium species (garlic, onions, leeks, and shallots); curcumins found in turmeric; and the flavonoids and monoterpenes found in the citrus family (orange, grapefruit, and lemon).

3. Some nutrients act as "suppressing agents." These agents work after the tissue has been exposed to a carcinogen by inhibiting the carcinogen's action or by suppressing the development of the cancer. Suppressing agents include: the protease inhibitors found in soybeans, benzyl isothiocyanates found in cabbage and broccoli, D-limonene found in oranges, vitamin

A found in carotene-rich fruits and vegetables, calcium found in leafy greens and dairy products, and the antioxidant nutrients found in orange and green fruits and vegetables.

4. Certain vitamins and minerals can strengthen the immune system that helps to protect the body from cancer. Vitamin A and the carotenoids, vitamin C, vitamin E, selenium, copper, zinc, and iron help the immune cells destroy viruses that may cause cancer.

5. The liver is capable of detoxifying, or making harmless, some carcinogens. A deficiency of certain nutrients will slow down this process of detoxification. Examples of this are riboflavin and pyridoxine (B-6) that are essential cofactors for a number of enzymes involved in detoxification. Unidentified components of the cruciferous vegetables may detoxify estrogens in the human body, making them less likely to promote breast cancer.

6. Some chemicals increase cell duplication rates, causing the cells to be more susceptible to cancer-causing agents. Phthalides and polyacetylenes, compounds found in carrots, celery, and parsley, regulate the manufacture of prostaglandin E-2, a compound that increases cell duplication rates. Other compounds found in garlic and onions also modulate prostaglandin synthesis. Calcium salts reduce cell duplication rates in the intestine.

DIETARY CHANGES
TO HELP PREVENT CANCER

1. Decrease the total amount of fat in your diet. Animals fed high-fat diets develop tumors of the mammary gland, intestinal tract, and pancreas more readily than those animals fed low-fat diets. A low-fat diet appears to prevent the promotion phase of cancer development.

2. Consume foods that are high in fiber. Fiber may help to reduce colon cancer. Insoluble fiber, the kind that is found in wheat bran and plant cell walls, may dilute a potential carcinogen by increasing fecal bulk. This reduces the exposure of the colon to a carcinogen. A high-fiber diet also reduces the time it takes for fecal material to pass through the colon, which also reduces exposure of the colon to carcinogens. Some studies also indicate that there may be a relationship between fiber and breast and stomach cancer. Diets rich in soluble fiber, including pectin and gums, found in fruits, vegetables, and some cereals, protect against these cancers but it is not known if this is due to the fiber or the presence or absence of another dietary component. Therefore it is wise to eat high-fiber foods and not rely on fiber supplements alone.

3. Eat foods that are rich in carotenoids. Smokers who rarely eat carotenoid-rich foods have a greater risk of cancer than smokers who eat one or more servings of these foods a day. The body can turn some of the carotenoids into vitamin A and vitamin A has been shown, in animals, to prevent, suppress, or retard some chemically induced cancers in the pancreas, prostate, lung, esophagus, and colon. Beta-carotene found in yellow and orange vegetables is associated with reduced risk of lung cancer and the lycopene found in tomatoes is an even stronger antioxidant.

4. Eat a diet rich in the antioxidant nutrients: vitamin E, selenium, the carotenoids, vitamin C, the flavonoids, and glutathione. Vitamin E and selenium may be related to an increased risk of some cancers such as breast and lung. Studies of large human populations suggest that vitamin C–containing foods may protect against cancer, particularly stomach cancer. Glutathione is a compound that is both an antioxidant and an anticarcinogen. It is present in high concentrations in oranges, cantaloupe, strawberries, fresh peaches, avocado, asparagus, squash, potatoes, okra, cauliflower, broccoli, and raw tomatoes.

5. Substitute soy products for some of the animal protein you eat. Soy products such as soymilk, soybeans, tofu, tempeh, and soycheese are low in saturated fat, cholesterol-free, and contain protease inhibitors that act as blocking agents.

6. Eat at least two servings of a vegetable from the cabbage family each day. These vegetables contain both blocking and suppressive agents.

7. Eat large amounts of garlic, onions, leeks, and shallots. These members of the Allium species contain several compounds that act as blocking and suppressive agents.

8. Eat one serving of a citrus fruit each day. Citrus fruits are sources of vitamin C, flavonoids, monoterpenes, and glutathione, compounds that act as blocking and suppressive agents.

9. Avoid salted, smoked, and pickled fish products as well as salted foods such as salt-cured ham, sausage, and salami. These foods have been linked to stomach cancer.

10. Do not charbroil meats and fish over an open flame. This can result in the formation of polycyclic hydrocarbons that are cancer initiators.

JUICES THAT MAY HELP
TO PREVENT CANCER

Broccoli: source of vitamin C, beta-carotene, indoles, glucobrassicin, glutathione, and isothiocyanates

Brussels sprouts: source of vitamin C, indoles, and isothiocyanates

Cabbage: source of vitamin C, indoles, isothiocyanates, and selenium

Cauliflower: source of vitamin C, indoles, isothiocyanates, and glutathione

Carrot: source of carotenoids, phthalides, and pro-vitamin A

Garlic, onions and leeks: source of organosulfur compounds

Orange: source of the monoterpenes, vitamin C, bioflavonoids, glutathione, and selenium

Kale: source of calcium, iron, beta-carotene, and indoles

Tomato: source of lycopene and glutathione

JUICE RECIPES

Apple Tea

Twice the taste but half the caffeine, this tea is a gentle stimulant to get you going in the morning. Green tea is a source of plant phenols that are cancer-blocking agents.

1 green tea bag
½ cup fresh apple juice

Brew tea in ½ cup boiling water. Add apple juice to tea and serve immediately.

Simply Orange

An antioxidant powerhouse, this juice is full of vitamin C, flavonoids, and selenium.

3 or 4 carrots, tops removed
2 oranges

Remove orange peel but not the white coat underneath (a source of bioflavonoids). Juice ingredients and garnish with a orange slice.

High-C Citrus Juice

Rich in vitamin C and flavonoids, this juice will help to boost your immune system.

1 orange
½ grapefruit
½ guava
crushed ice

Remove the peel from orange and grapefruit but not the white coat underneath. Juice all ingredients. Pour over ice, garnish with an orange slice, and serve immediately.

Coleslaw in a Glass

A tasty blend of cancer blockers and suppressors. This drink may help prevent breast cancer.

¼ head green cabbage
1 carrot, top removed
1 thin onion slice

Juice all ingredients and garnish with a carrot curl.

Carotene Cocktail

This drink contains a blend of the antioxidant carotenoids.

1 tomato
2 carrots, tops removed
1 collard leaf

Juice ingredients. Garnish with a cherry tomato.

Sweet Cabbage Juice

A drink for those who think that cabbage juice couldn't possibly taste great.

2 round slices pineapple
¼ head cabbage

Prepare pineapple according to the directions that came with your juicer. Juice ingredients and garnish with a wedge of pineapple.

Hot Tomato

Try this juice if you like spicy hot food. It's guaranteed to clear your head.

3 medium tomatoes
1 clove garlic, peeled
¼-inch slice hot red pepper

Juice all ingredients and serve immediately.

Brassica Tonic

A mixture of veggies from the Brassica (cabbage) family. Loaded with cancer blockers and suppressors as well as vitamin C and beta-carotene.

2 stalks celery, leaves trimmed
1 kale leaf
1 broccoli spear
1 wedge green cabbage

Save celery leaves for a salad and juice rest of ingredients. Garnish with a small celery stalk.

Smiling Tomato

The taste of sweet onion in this juice will bring a smile to your face.

1 medium tomato
1 medium cucumber
1 thin slice sweet onion

Peel cucumber if it is not organic. Juice ingredients and garnish with a slice of cucumber.

Garden Cooler

This juice is rich in lycopene, beta-carotene, and vitamin C.

4 Brussels sprouts
1 tomato
½ sweet pepper
lime wedge
crushed ice

Follow your juicer's instructions for juicing limes. Juice ingredients and pour over ice. Garnish with a twist of lime and serve immediately.

CHAPTER FIVE

Hypertension

High blood pressure or hypertension affects one out of every ten people and it has been estimated that thirty to forty million Americans suffer from this condition. Overweight individuals, African-Americans, and people who do not exercise are at greater risk for developing this disorder. Hypertension is not a disease, it does not kill people directly. Rather it contributes to death rates by aggravating cardiac heart disease or by initiating a stroke.

WHAT IS HYPERTENSION?

When blood is propelled through the arteries by the heart, it pushes on the walls of the arteries with a measurable force. This force is called blood pressure. Blood pressure is measured at two readings. The first is the *systolic blood pressure* (SBP), which is taken when the ventricles of the heart are contracting and pushing blood into the arteries. The second is the *diastolic blood pressure* (DBP), which is taken when the ventricles are relaxed. The diastolic pressure represents the lowest pressure that is placed upon the arterial walls and it is the pressure most useful in evaluating an individual's risk for heart disease or stroke. The classification of blood pressure most commonly used is that published in 1978 by the World Health Organization Expert Committee:

Normal blood pressure: SBP is less than or equal to 140 mm Hg and DBP is less than or equal to 90 mm Hg.
Borderline hypertension: SBP is between 141 and 159 mm Hg and DBP is between 91 and 94 mm Hg.
Hypertension: SBP is greater than or equal to 160 mm Hg or DBP is greater than or equal to 95 mm Hg.

WHAT CAUSES HYPERTENSION?

Hypertension is a disorder with many different causes. Factors that influence blood pressure include: the resistance of blood flow in the vessels, the pumping action of the heart, the thickness of the blood, the elasticity of the arteries, and the amount of blood in the vascular system. Some individuals inherit a tendency to hypertension that remains dormant until something in the environment triggers an unknown mechanism that raises blood pressure.

HOW DIET CAN HELP
TO PREVENT HYPERTENSION

Rates of hypertension are lowest in societies where the individuals are physically active, lean vegetarians who do not drink alcohol. Rates of hypertension are highest among societies with a sedentary lifestyle, who consume a diet high in calories, fat, alcohol, and salt and low in potassium. Which part of the vegetarian diet protects against hypertension? Below are some of the major theories.

1. People living in remote villages in areas of Asia, Africa, and South America who naturally eat a low-salt diet rarely develop high blood pressure. However, when some of these people move to coastal areas where a high-sodium diet is consumed, their chance of developing hypertension increases. It is thought that in some people the kidney is unable to excrete normal amounts of sodium at normal blood pressure. The body responds by increasing the pressure until sodium excretion matches sodium intake. These individuals will be able to keep their blood pressure normal by following a low-sodium diet.

2. Some researchers believe that primitive societies have a low incidence of hypertension not because of their low-sodium intake, but because of their high potassium intake. They think that for some individuals to maintain normal blood pressure they must eat more potassium than sodium. (This is called a low sodium to potassium ratio.)

3. The minerals magnesium and calcium have also been shown to lower blood pressure. Magnesium relaxes the muscle cells in arteries by regulating calcium. Calcium may help to regulate sodium levels inside cells. High dietary sodium levels in turn can increase the loss of calcium from the kidney. The actions of these minerals are interrelated and so it is wise to include generous amounts of both minerals in your diet.

4. Consuming too many calories in the form of fat and carbohydrate has been shown to stimulate the sympathetic nervous system, which causes the muscles in the arteries to tighten and the heart rate to increase. These factors elevate blood pressure. The pattern in which the fat is stored is important as well. Individuals who have excess weight distributed mainly in the upper part of the body and waist are more prone to develop hypertension than individuals who store fat in the buttocks and thighs.

DIETARY CHANGES
TO PREVENT HYPERTENSION

1. Decrease the amount of salt in your diet. Take the salt shaker off your table and do not add salt to the water you cook vegetables in (steam them instead). Season vegetables with herbs and lemon juice. Avoid salted snacks such as potato chips, crackers, and pretzels.

2. Increase the amount of potassium-rich foods in your diet. This mineral has lowered blood pressure in individuals with high blood pressure and in individuals with normal pressure. Potassium rich foods include: nuts, avocado, leafy green vegetables, beans, broccoli, yams, and bananas.

3. Make sure you are getting enough calcium each day. This mineral is involved in the regulation of many bodily processes that can influence blood pressure and some studies have shown that a diet rich in calcium helps to lower blood pressure. Good sources of calcium include: nonfat dairy products, calcium-fortified soymilk, tofu, corn tortillas, collard leaves, turnip greens, and broccoli. CAUTION: Although spinach, Swiss chard, and beet greens are often recommended as calcium sources, these greens contain oxalates that bind the calcium, making it unavailable to the body. This is especially true for their juices, which may react with other calcium sources in your stomach to reduce the total amount of calcium you absorb from the meal.

4. Eat a diet rich in magnesium. Like calcium, this mineral is involved in many processes that could influence blood pressure. Some studies have indicated that low magnesium levels may be associated with high blood pressure. Foods that are good sources of magnesium include: nuts, brewer's yeast, soybeans, dried apricots, collard leaves, and whole grain breads.

5. Eat at least two vitamin C–rich foods each day. This vitamin has been shown in several studies to lower blood pressure. The mechanism responsible has not been identified. Vitamin C–rich foods include: sweet peppers, vegetables in the cabbage family, and fruits in the citrus family.

6. Serve fish three or four times a week. Fish oil, added to a low salt diet, decreases blood pressure better than fish oil alone. This may be because the omega-3 fatty acids in fish purge the body of excess salt. Sources of fish oil include: herring, mackerel, halibut, lake trout, whitefish, and salmon. If you decide to take fish oil supplements, always take your capsules with fish to increase their effectiveness.

7. Eliminate or greatly reduce your alcohol intake. In the United States it has been estimated that 10 percent of middle-aged men have hypertension because of excess alcohol.

JUICES TO HELP PREVENT
HYPERTENSION

Broccoli: source of calcium, magnesium, and vitamin C
Cantaloupe: source of potassium
Carrot: source of potassium and magnesium
Celery: source of potassium and magnesium
Collard leaves: source of magnesium, calcium, potassium, and vitamin C
Kale: source of calcium and vitamin C
Lettuce: source of potassium
Orange: source of vitamin C and potassium
Papaya: source of potassium
Tomato: source of potassium and vitamin C

JUICE RECIPES

Creamy Orange Shake

This shake is rich in calcium, magnesium, and potassium

3 oranges, peeled
½ cup nonfat plain yogurt
1 ripe banana, peeled
1 teaspoon brewer's yeast (optional)

Juice oranges and combine juice with yogurt, yeast, and banana in a blender. Process until smooth. Pour into a glass and garnish with an orange twist.

Potassium Snap

About 1½ grams of potassium are packed into this juice combination.

½ cantaloupe
½-inch slice ginger root
1 ripe banana, peeled

Prepare cantaloupe according to your juicer's instructions. Juice cantaloupe and ginger. Add juice to blender with banana and process until smooth.

Veggie Mineral Cooler

This drink is high in calcium, magnesium, and potassium.

1 collard leaf
3 stalks celery, leaves trimmed
1 spear broccoli
½ cucumber, peeled

Juice ingredients and garnish with a small celery stalk.

Triple Leaf Juice

A combination of juices that is high in beta-carotene, calcium, and vitamin C.

1 collard leaf
1 kale leaf
2 lettuce leaves
1 cucumber

If cucumber is waxed or not organic, remove peel. Juice ingredients and garnish with an asparagus spear.

Green Calcium Drink

This drink is high in calcium, magnesium, and potassium.

2 kale leaves
2 carrots, tops removed
2 broccoli spears

Juice vegetables. Garnish with a carrot curl and serve.

Brassica Tonic

A mixture of veggies from the Brassica (cabbage) family. Loaded with cancer blockers and suppressors.

2 stalks celery, leaves trimmed
1 kale leaf
1 broccoli spear
1 wedge green cabbage

Save celery leaves for a salad and juice rest of ingredients. Garnish with a small celery stalk.

Red Calcium Drink

Another juice that is high in calcium, potassium, and magnesium.

3 medium tomatoes
2 large kale leaves

Juice ingredients and garnish with a cherry tomato.

Special K Cooler

This icy drink is mineral rich.

cucumber juice, frozen into cubes
2 cucumbers, peeled
1 kale leaf

Juice cucumbers and kale and pour over frozen juice cubes.

Carotene Cocktail

This drink contains a blend of the antioxidant carotenoids.

1 tomato
2 carrots, tops removed
1 collard leaf

Juice ingredients. Garnish with a cherry tomato.

Summer Splash

This is a potassium-rich drink that will replenish minerals lost through exercise.

2 stalks celery
½ papaya, peeled
½ cup ice water

Juice celery and papaya. Mix juice with ice water and serve.

Tomato Zinger

Rich in beta-carotene and potassium.

1 leaf red cabbage
3 tomatoes
1 stalk celery

Juice vegetables, garnish with a cherry tomato, and serve immediately.

Celery Cooler

This drink stores well without loss of taste or minerals. Store it in a thermos and bring to work or school.

2 stalks celery
4 oranges, peeled

Rinse thermos with cold water and place in freezer overnight. Juice ingredients and pour into prepared thermos.

Hypertension Tonic

An eight-ounce glass of this juice contains about 1,000 milligrams of potassium.

⅓ cantaloupe
2 stalks celery

Prepare cantaloupe according to the directions of your juicer. Juice ingredients and serve immediately.

Caesar Salad in a Glass

Rich in potassium, this juice is a pressure reliever.

4 leaves Romaine lettuce
2 stalks celery
¼ lemon
1 clove garlic

Juice all ingredients and serve immediately.

CHAPTER SIX

Stroke

In the United States, stroke is the third leading cause of death. The American Heart Association estimates that 1.87 million people in the United States had strokes in 1983. Fifteen percent of these people died from the stroke, 16 percent had to be put in health-care facilities and 50 percent were permanently disabled. Your chances of having a stroke are very low until you reach the age of 45, after which they rise rapidly, more than doubling each decade.

WHAT IS A STROKE?

The cells of the brain need blood to supply them with oxygen and glucose. A stroke or *cerebral vascular accident* (CVA) occurs when this blood supply is abruptly reduced or stopped, resulting in damage to the brain cells. If a CVA is severe, weakness or paralysis may occur in one half of the body, the victim may forget how to speak or lose muscular coordination. If the blood supply is temporarily reduced, but not totally lost, tissue damage is not permanent and the victim experiences a brief blackout, blurred vision, or dizziness. This is called a *transient ischemic attack* (TIA). A TIA is an important warning sign that blood flow in the brain is threatened.

WHAT CAUSES STROKE?

In the United States, the leading cause of stroke is a blockage by a blood clot in an artery narrowed by atherosclerosis. In other words, a stroke is the brain's version of a heart attack. A stroke can also be caused by a leakage of blood from the arteries into the brain tissue as a result of a burst artery. Arteries become brittle with age and if the blood pressure rises above normal this can lead to a break in the artery. The most common site for hemorrhage is near the motor nerves that control the face, arms, and legs. A hemorrhage that kills these cells will leave the victim partially paralyzed.

HOW DIET CAN HELP
TO PREVENT STROKE

Strokes that are caused by hemorrhage are more common among individuals who have high blood pressure. A diet that contains nutrients that lower blood pressure will also lower your chance of having this kind of stroke. A stroke that is caused by a blood clot is more common among individuals who have coronary heart disease, since they are both the result of atherosclerosis. A diet that reduces coronary heart disease (CHD) will also reduce your chances of having this kind of stroke.

DIETARY CHANGES TO PREVENT STROKE

1. Greatly reduce or eliminate sources of saturated fat and cholesterol from your diet. You can accomplish this by eating no more than one three-ounce serving of animal flesh each day. At least three times a week this serving should be cold water fish, including: salmon, halibut, lake trout, herring, mackerel, and whitefish. Eat red meat no more than twice a week, choosing only lean cuts that are not cured or smoked. Remove the skin from poultry. By decreasing the amount of saturated fat and cholesterol in your diet, you can decrease the amount of cholesterol in your blood. Eating fish will help to keep blood pressure down and your blood less likely to clot.

2. Consume only nonfat dairy products. Whole milk and whole milk products are a significant source of cholesterol and saturated fat. Replace these fatty foods with their low or nonfat counterpart. Dairy products include: milk, cheese, yogurt, ice cream, and other frozen desserts.

3. Include a serving of soyfoods in your daily diet. In some people this may help to lower cholesterol levels. Soy products include: soybeans, tofu, tempeh, and calcium-fortified soymilk. Consider substituting fortified soymilk for cow's milk.

4. Eat at least three servings of calcium rich leafy green vegetables a day. These include: collard leaves, turnips greens, broccoli, kale, and Chinese cabbage. These greens are also rich in magnesium, potassium, and other minerals that may lower blood pressure. Remember, spinach, Swiss chard, beet greens, and the juices made from them, are *not* calcium sources and may actually lower the total calcium absorbed from meals they are part of.

5. Eat foods high in soluble fiber. Soluble fiber acts as a sponge in the intestine, soaking up cholesterol and preventing the body from reabsorbing and recycling it. Foods that contain soluble fiber include all fruits and vegetables, oats, and psyllium seed.

6. Eat at least two servings of a vitamin C–rich food each day. Vitamin C will help to prevent free radical damage to the arteries in your brain as well as lower blood pressure. Vitamin C–rich foods include: sweet peppers, vegetables in the cabbage family (cabbage, kale, broccoli), and fruits in the citrus family.

7. Eat liberal amounts of onions, garlic, cantaloupe, and ginger. These foods are natural blood thinners. Onions and garlic will also aid in lowering blood pressure.

8. Eat foods rich in vitamin E, beta-carotene, and other antioxidants. They will help to protect the arteries in your brain from free radical damage. Sunflower seeds, almonds, olive oil, and wheat germ are good sources of vitamin E. Orange-fleshed fruits such as papaya and cantaloupe, orange and yellow colored vegetables such as carrots and sweet potatoes, and leafy green vegetables such as kale and collards are good sources of beta-carotene.

JUICES TO PREVENT STROKE

Asparagus: source of vitamin E and beta-carotene

Bok choy (Chinese cabbage): source of calcium, vitamin C, and beta-carotene

Broccoli: source of carotenoids, vitamin C, calcium, and potassium

Cantaloupe: source of a natural blood thinner

Carrot: source of beta-carotene, copper, and selenium

Celery: source of potassium and magnesium

Collard greens: source of calcium, magnesium, potassium, beta-carotene, and vitamin C

Garlic: source of a natural blood thinner and cholesterol-lowering agent

Ginger: source of natural blood thinner

Orange: source of selenium, vitamin C, and flavonoids

JUICE RECIPES

Calcium Cooler

This drink is a good source of calcium, beta-carotene, and the other carotenoids.

¼ head Chinese cabbage (bok choy)
6 carrots, tops removed

Juice vegetables. Garnish with a carrot curl and serve immediately.

Summer Delight

This combination is thirst quenching and full of blood thinners.

¼ cantaloupe
1-inch round slice of watermelon
½ orange, peeled
crushed ice

Prepare melons according to your juicer's directions. Juice fruit and pour juices over ice, shake briefly to cool, and pour into tall glasses while straining out ice.

Purplepower

Contains a natural blood thinner.

2 large bunches seeded red grapes
½-inch slice ginger root

Prepare grapes according to your juicer's directions. Juice fruit and ginger. Pour into a tall glass and garnish with a small bunch of grapes.

Garlic Lovers Tonic

This powerful juice is rich in calcium, carotenes, and ajoene.

¼ head bok choy (Chinese cabbage)
5 carrots, tops removed
2 cloves garlic, peeled
2 stalks celery

Juice vegetables. Serve immediately.

Heart Happy Veggie Drink

This drink contains ajoene, a natural blood thinner, as well as all the antioxidants.

1 garlic clove
3 carrots, tops removed
1 kale leaf
2 spears asparagus

Juice ingredients and drink immediately.

Potassium Snap

This drink contains about 1½ grams of potassium.

½ cantaloupe
½-inch slice ginger root
1 ripe banana, peeled

Prepare cantaloupe according to your juicer's instructions. Juice cantaloupe and ginger. Add juice to blender with banana and process until smooth.

Pink Power Veggie Drink

This drink will keep your heart in the pink. It contains a blood thinner and is loaded with vitamin C and beta-carotene.

1 sweet red pepper
¼ small onion
3 carrots, tops removed

Juice ingredients and garnish with a carrot curl and slice of red pepper.

Onion Salad Splash

Use this juice instead of fat-laden dressings on salads or as a seasoning for vegetables.

3 or 4 lemons
½ onion

Prepare lemons according to your juicer's instructions. Juice ingredients and store in refrigerator. Shake before using.

Tropical Snowstorm

Spicy and cold, this drink contains a natural blood thinner as well as vitamin C.

two 1-inch-round slices pineapple
1-inch slice ginger root
¼ guava
crushed ice

Fill tall glass with crushed ice and place in freezer until glass is frosted. Prepare pineapple according to your juicer's instructions. Juice fruit and ginger, pour into frozen glass, and serve with a straw and pineapple spear.

CHAPTER SEVEN

Noninsulin Dependent Diabetes Mellitus

Diabetes is the seventh leading cause of death in the United States. In 1982, diabetes was identified as the underlying cause of almost 35,000 deaths in this country and it was listed as the contributing cause in an additional 95,000 deaths. Noninsulin dependent diabetes mellitus (NIDDM), sometimes called adult onset diabetes or type II diabetes, affects about 90 percent of the individuals who are diabetics. In the years 1935 and 1936, NIDDM was present in 3.8 per 10,000 people. By the period 1979 to 1981, this rate had risen to 22.7 per 10,000 people. Approximately 9 percent of people 65 years old and older are believed to have NIDDM. Fortunately, not only is this type of diabetes largely preventable, it is almost 100 percent reversible with a proper diet and medication.

WHAT IS NIDDM?

Glucose is one of the main fuels that the body uses to provide energy. The central nervous system uses about nine tablespoons of glucose each day while the red blood cells need about three tablespoons of glucose. Glucose is the only form of carbohydrate that can be transported by the blood to all the tissues, including the skeletal muscles, heart and lungs. At any one time, the body keeps 100 milligrams of glucose per 100 ml (or deciliter) of blood. Whenever the amount of glucose in the blood rises above 160 milligrams/deciliter, a person is said to have too much sugar in his blood or *hyperglycemia*. This occurs when the pancreas does not secrete enough of the hormone insulin or when the cells of the body become resistant to insulin. On a cellular level, glucose cannot penetrate a cell's membrane without insulin. When insulin is present, glucose leaves the blood and is able to enter the hungry cells. The kidneys usually reabsorb the glucose that flows through them; however, when glucose levels get too high, the kidneys cannot keep up and sugar "spills" into the urine. The loss of glucose causes a greater production of urine. To replace lost fluids your body triggers its "thirst" mechanism. Therefore the symptoms of diabetes are: high blood glucose, glucose in the urine, excessive thirst, and frequent urination.

WHAT CAUSES NIDDM?

At the cell membrane, glucose pairs with a carrier substance that transports it through the membrane and releases it inside the cell. This transport will only take place if insulin is attached to the insulin receptor site on the cell's surface. Some people do not have enough insulin receptors or the receptors are some-how defective. This is called *insulin resistance:* insulin is present but it cannot be used by the cell. Insulin is secreted by the beta cells of the islets of Langerhans in the pancreas. As we age, the amount of insulin se-creted by the beta cells gradually decreases. The only way for our bodies to manage with this reduced level of hormone is to decrease requirements by eating less. A combination of decreased quantities of insulin with increased insulin resistance causes type II diabetes.

HOW DIET CAN HELP
TO PREVENT NIDDM

A proper diet can help increase glucose sensitivity (decrease resistance) and decrease weight, a high risk factor for NIDDM. Mild forms of NIDDM can sometimes be totally controlled by diet.

1. Some nutrients help prevent diabetes. Popula-tions that eat large amounts of fruit, vegetables, and unrefined foods have a lower incidence of diabetes. Many researchers believe this is because of the fiber content of whole grains, fruits, and vegetables. Solu-ble fiber is found in oats, apples, carrots, beans, and lentils. Insoluble fiber is found in all fruits and vegetables and wheat bran. Insoluble fiber slows down the release of carbohydrate into the blood, preventing hyperglycemia.

2. Some dietary changes can decrease insulin resist-ance by increasing the sensitivity of the cell mem-brane to glucose. These changes include: eating a diet that is low in total fat; consuming more cold water fish such as mackerel, herring, salmon, whitefish, lake trout, and halibut; and eating foods high in the mineral chromium and insulin promoting factor. A moderate weight loss will also increase glucose sensi-

tivity. An obese person may only have to lose twenty or thirty pounds to enjoy this benefit.

3. Some dietary changes, such as a low-fat diet or high intake of vitamin C, can reduce glucose production in the liver.

THE DIABETES PREVENTION DIET

1. Choose foods that are whole and unrefined. High-fiber diets may protect genetically prone individuals from developing diabetes. Foods that contain fiber are: all fruits and vegetables, beans and lentils, seeds and nuts, and whole grains.

2. Eliminate high-fat foods and substitute their low-fat versions. A low-fat diet will keep the liver from increasing its production of glucose, decrease insulin resistance, and lower weight. Some foods that contain fat are: all whole milk products, all fats and oils including mayonnaise and salad dressing, fatty muscle meats, poultry skin, and fried foods.

3. Consume foods that are rich in chromium. This mineral is an essential trace element needed for normal carbohydrate metabolism. Foods that contain chromium: apples, barley, and other whole grains; brewer's yeast; and acidic foods that have contact with stainless steel.

4. Eat a diet rich in manganese. This trace mineral is involved in many facets of carbohydrate metabolism.

5. Reduce alcohol consumption. In animals and humans, administration of large doses of alcohol after meals results in high blood sugar.

6. Include vitamin C–rich foods in your daily diet.
Vitamin C will help to keep glucose production by the
liver at normal levels. Sources of vitamin C: sweet
peppers, citrus fruits, strawberries, cabbage, broccoli,
and kale.

7. Eat foods that are high in insulin promoting factor.
These foods and spices have been shown to increase
glucose tolerance. Sources of insulin promoting factor: tuna, peanut butter, cloves, bay leaves, apple pie
spice, cinnamon, and turmeric.

**8. Eat a three-ounce serving of fish three or four times a
week.** Dutch researchers at the National Institute of
Public Health found that one ounce of fish (lean, fatty,
or canned), protects against the development of glucose intolerance, a condition that often foreshadows
diabetes.

JUICES TO HELP PREVENT
TYPE II DIABETES

Apple: source of pectin and chromium
Brussels sprouts: source of manganese and vitamin C
Cabbage: source of manganese, chromium, and vita-
min C
Ginger: alcohol replacement, adds "zip" to nonalco-
holic drinks
Green pepper: source of vitamin C and chromium
Kale: source of vitamin C
Spinach: source of manganese, chromium, and vita-
min C
Strawberries: source of vitamin C
Sweet peppers: source of chromium and vitamin C
Turnip greens: source of manganese and vitamin C

JUICE RECIPES

Brussels Hop

This is a manganese and vitamin C–rich drink.

8 Brussels sprouts
8 carrots, tops removed
¼ apple, cored

Juice ingredients. Garnish with a carrot curl and serve immediately.

Ginger Fizz

A great drink with natural energy sources guaranteed to make you the life of the party.

½ inch slice ginger root
½ grapefruit, peeled
½ tart apple, cored
sparkling water
ice cubes

Juice ginger and fruit. Pour over ice and add sparkling water. Garnish with twist of orange.

Chromium Special

This drink is high in chromium, manganese, and vitamin C.

¼ head green cabbage
1 green pepper
1 small bunch spinach

Juice vegetables. Garnish with a small spinach leaf and serve immediately.

Super Chromium Shake

This shake is high in chromium, vitamin C, and the B-complex vitamins.

1 orange, peeled
1 cup strawberries
1 ripe banana, peeled
1 heaping tablespoon brewer's yeast

Remove green caps from strawberries and juice berries and orange. Combine juice, banana, and yeast in blender and process until smooth.

Cinnamon Shake

This is a fiber-rich shake that contains an insulin-promoting factor as well as chromium.

1 apple, cored
½ teaspoon cinnamon
1 ripe banana, peeled
½ cup fortified soymilk

Juice apple. In a blender combine juice with remaining ingredients and process until smooth. Pour into a glass. Sprinkle cinnamon on top and serve immediately.

Summer Sparkler

A low-sugar alternative to soda pop.

1 grapefruit, peeled
1 apple, cored
sparkling water
crushed ice

Juice fruit and pour into tall, ice filled glass. Add sparkling water.

Apple Pie in a Cup

A warm, friendly spicy drink that will supply your body with chromium and other insulin promoting factors.

4 apples
¼-inch slice ginger root
¼ teaspoon apple pie spice

Remove seeds from apples and juice apples and ginger. In a saucepan or microwave, combine spice and juice and gently warm. Serve in a mug.

Manganese Tonic

This drink is rich in the mineral manganese as well as vitamin C.

¼ head of green cabbage
4 Brussels sprouts
1 turnip green

Juice ingredients and serve immediately.

Calcium Tonic

This tonic will provide your body with the minerals calcium, magnesium, and manganese.

2 turnip leaves
1 collard leaf
6 carrots, tops removed

Juice vegetables. Garnish with a carrot curl and serve immediately.

Triple Leaf Juice

This juice is high in beta-carotene, calcium, and vitamin C.

1 collard leaf
1 kale leaf
2 lettuce leaves
1 cucumber

If cucumber is waxed or not organic, remove peel. Juice ingredients and garnish with an asparagus spear.

CHAPTER EIGHT

Osteoporosis

About fifteen million people in the United States suffer from osteoporosis, causing approximately 1.3 million fractures of the vertebrae, hips, forearms, and other bones each year. Both sexes are affected, but the bone loss is greater in women than in men because of hormone loss during menopause. Approximately 20 percent of women in the United States suffer one or more fractures caused by osteoporosis by age 65 and as many as 40 percent experience fractures after the age of 65.

WHAT IS OSTEOPOROSIS?

Bone is made of calcium, phosphorus, magnesium, and various other trace minerals, embedded in an organic matrix of collagen and osteocalcin. Compact or cortical bone forms the main structural support of long bones, and spongy or trabecular bone provides elasticity as well as strength to the ends of bones and the vertebrae of the spine. Osteoporosis occurs when the amount of bone decreases. The bone that is present is normal in every way, it is just too low in mass to mechanically support the body. Type I osteoporosis is a bone loss in the trabecular (spongy) bone. It usually afflicts postmenopausal women between the ages of 51 and 65 years and is associated with estrogen loss. These women often experience fractures in the vertebrae of the neck. Type II osteoporosis occurs in a large proportion of women or men who are more than 75 years old. It is characterized by a loss of spongy and compact bone and most often results in hip fractures.

WHAT CAUSES OSTEOPOROSIS?

Although we tend to think of bones as solid blocks of minerals, they are actually composed of living, breathing cells: the osteoblasts, osteoclasts, and osteocytes. Osteoclasts and osteocytes are constantly forming new bone while the osteoblasts are constantly resorbing old bone. Usually these two opposite forces equal each other in adult life. However under some circumstances, bone loss is greater than bone formation and a decrease in bone mass occurs. Estrogen loss, lack of exercise, lack of calcium, and a decreased ability to absorb nutrients all play a role in this imbalance of bone metabolism.

HOW DIET CAN HELP
TO PREVENT OSTEOPOROSIS

Prevention of osteoporosis depends upon three factors: hormone therapy, exercise, and diet. Dietary supplementation works best when combined with either exercise or hormone replacement therapy. This may be especially true for type I osteoporosis. Your diet can help in six ways.

1. Building bone mass in your young adult years may help to prevent bone loss. This can be done by eating a diet that supplies adequate minerals for bone production. Calcium, magnesium, and phosphorus are the main minerals needed for bone formation, but the trace minerals boron and zinc may also be important.

2. Bone is not composed of minerals alone. The nutrients necessary for the development and maintenance of the organic matrix must also be present. These include vitamin K and vitamin C.

3. Absorption of vitamins and minerals necessary for bone formation decreases in senior years. Extra calcium may be needed to overcome absorption deficiencies. Antacids containing aluminum will decrease calcium absorption.

4. The kidneys are responsible for converting vitamin D into its active form and this function decreases with age. In addition, vitamin D synthesis in the skin also decreases with age. This vitamin is necessary for proper calcium metabolism.

5. Some foods increase the loss of calcium in the urine. For example, high animal-protein diets or high-phosphate diets are suspected of doing this.

6. Increased bone reabsorption may be the result of high salt diets. Sodium may compete with calcium for reabsorption in the kidney tubules and salt can increase parathyroid hormone levels that may elevate blood pressure and increase bone reabsorption.

DIETARY RECOMMENDATIONS
TO PREVENT OSTEOPOROSIS

1. Increase the calcium content of your diet. Good sources of calcium are: nonfat dairy products, calcium-fortified soymilk, tofu, corn tortillas, collard leaves, turnip greens, kale, and broccoli. CAUTION: Spinach, Swiss chard, and beet greens are not calcium sources and can decrease the amount of calcium you absorb for any meal they are eaten with. This is especially true for their juices.

2. Increase foods that are high in magnesium. This mineral is found in all green vegetables, particularly leafy greens, as well as tofu, nuts, and soybeans.

3. Substitute soyfoods for meat and dairy products. This will lower animal-protein and phosphate levels that are associated with calcium losses in the urine. Vegetarians have a lower incidence of osteoporosis than nonvegetarians. Soyfoods include: tofu, soymilk, soybeans, tempeh, and soycheese.

4. If you do not drink milk or fortified soymilk, consider taking a vitamin D supplement. This is especially important if you rarely get out of doors or if you live in an area that receives little sunlight.

5. Increase your consumption of bok choy, collards, kale, and turnip greens. These vegetables are sources of vitamin K, vitamin C and boron, nutrients needed to build a strong matrix.

6. Decrease the salt content of your diet. A high salt diet may increase the loss of calcium in the urine.

7. Eliminate soft drinks and substitute juice drinks. Soft drinks are high in phosphates that increase calcium loss in animal studies.

8. Decrease the amount of caffeine and alcohol you drink. Daily consumption of two and one half cups of coffee a day increases the risk of hip fractures. Women who drink more than one ounce of alcohol a day were more likely to suffer forearm and hip fractures.

9. Increase foods that are high in copper and zinc. These minerals are also important in bone health. Copper sources include: oysters, nuts, soy lecithin, split peas, peanuts, and cod liver oil. Zinc sources include: oysters, ginger root, nuts, split peas, whole grains, chicken, and clams.

JUICES TO PREVENT OSTEOPOROSIS

Broccoli: source of calcium, vitamin C, vitamin K, and magnesium
Bok choy (Chinese cabbage): source of vitamin C and calcium
Carrot: source of zinc and copper
Collards: source of calcium, vitamin C, vitamin K, magnesium, and boron
Garlic: source of copper and zinc
Ginger: source of zinc and substitute for alcohol
Kale: source of calcium, vitamin C, vitamin K, magnesium, and boron
Lemon: source of vitamin C, and a salt substitute
Orange: source of vitamin C
Papaya: source of vitamin C and copper
Turnip greens: source of calcium, vitamin C, vitamin K, magnesium, and boron

JUICE RECIPES

Papaya Shake

A calcium and vitamin C–rich drink that will make your bones give a sigh of relief.

1 papaya
½ cup fortified soymilk
1 banana, peeled
1 teaspoon vanilla extract

Prepare papaya according to your juicer's instructions. Combine juice and other ingredients in blender. Process until smooth and serve immediately.

Citrus Chocolate Cooler

A calcium-rich drink for chocolate lovers.

2 oranges
1 wedge lime
4 ounces fortified chocolate soymilk

Peel fruit and juice. Mix juice with soymilk and pour into glasses. Garnish with a slice of orange.

Green Calcium Drink

This drink is high in calcium, magnesium, and potassium.

2 kale leaves
2 carrots, tops removed
2 broccoli spears

Juice vegetables. Garnish with a carrot curl and serve.

Six-Veggie Calcium Tonic

Rich in calcium, magnesium, vitamin K, vitamin C, and all the bone-building nutrients.

4 or 5 carrots, tops removed
1 kale leaf
1 broccoli spear
2 leaves bok choy
½ cucumber

Peel cucumber if it is not organic or if it is waxed. Juice vegetables, pour into glass and drink immediately.

Four-Veggie Calcium Tonic

Another great bone-builder rich in vitamin C and calcium.

2 tomatoes
½ red pepper
¼ head bok choy
½ small rutabaga

Juice vegetables and serve immediately.

Hawaiian Snowstorm

The tropical way to get your vitamin C and trace minerals.

fresh orange juice
1 papaya
one 2-inch slice pineapple
¼-inch ginger root

Dilute orange juice with water and freeze. Crush frozen juice and spoon into glass. Prepare pineapple and papaya according to your juicer's instructions. Juice fruit and ginger root and pour juice over ice in a tall glass.

Brassica Tonic

A mixture of veggies from the Brassica (cabbage) family. Loaded with cancer blockers and suppressors.

2 stalks celery, leaves trimmed
1 kale leaf
1 broccoli spear
1 wedge green cabbage

Juice all ingredients. Garnish with a small celery stalk.

The OK Special

The benefits of vegetable juice with a taste like fruit juice. Rich in vitamin C and folacin.

3 oranges, peeled
1 kale leaf

Juice ingredients and serve immediately.

CHAPTER NINE

Immune Enhancement

Our bodies are constantly under attack from the viruses, bacteria, and parasites that surround us on the outside and potentially cancerous cells that develop on the inside. We survive these threats and even flourish because of the constant surveillance of our immune system. Keeping our immune system in optimal fighting condition is one of the best ways we can prevent infectious diseases.

WHAT IS THE IMMUNE SYSTEM?

The immune system is one of the most complicated systems of the body. It is composed of the cells of the thymus, lymph nodes, spleen, and bone marrow and has no central organ of control. Its cells patrol the organs of the body using the circulatory system and lymph vessels as highways. When bacteria or viruses enter the body, the immune system reacts in two ways: the humoral response and the cell-mediated response. The humoral response involves the production of antibodies specifically designed to react with a microbe. The cell-mediated response is not as specific. These cells attack and engulf anything that they recognize as "nonself."

HOW DOES THE
IMMUNE SYSTEM WORK?

The immune response is extremely complicated and intricate. Below is a very basic explanation of what happens when the body is invaded by a virus or bacteria.

The first immune cells to arrive when a microbe is detected are neutrophils. These white blood cells start to eat (phagocytize) the microbes while sending a signal to another type of white cell, the macrophages, that an invader is present. When the macrophages arrive they process the antigens on the surface of the bacteria and present them to the B-lymphocyte cells that manufacture antibodies to attack the microbes. The antibodies are capable of traveling throughout the body in the blood, attacking any of the now rapidly multiplying bacteria wherever they may be hiding. Macrophages also secrete chemicals (interferons, interleukins, and prostaglandins) that communicate with other immune cells. Another group of lymphocytes are the T lymphocytes or *T*-cells. T-cells, along with other immune cells including the natural killer (NK) cells, do not manufacture antibodies but instead recognize cells as invaders by recognizing that they are nonself. They protect against not only viral and bacterial infection but also tumor growth.

HOW DIET CAN ENHANCE IMMUNE FUNCTION

The immune system can suffer when the body lacks nutrients due to a poor diet, loss of nutrients during stress, or malnutrition due to alcoholism. It can take longer to perform its job and may eventually require the use of antibiotics to destroy the bacteria or virus. The following nutrients are necessary for a well-nourished, optimally active immune system.

Iron

A decreased resistance to infections is found in iron-deficient children. They show abnormalities in the function of the lymphocytes and neutrophils.

Protein

Individuals who do not eat enough protein have reduced immune function. Although protein deficiency is rare in the United States, it can occur during periods of prolonged illness or due to loss of appetite in the elderly.

Zinc

Supplementation with this mineral stimulates the immune system. Zinc levels are often low in the elderly, leading to susceptibility to infections.

Copper

This trace mineral is necessary for the immune system to function properly although its exact role in the process is not yet known.

Selenium

This trace mineral is a cofactor of glutathione peroxidase, an enzyme involved in cellular antioxidation. It is also involved in antibody production and protects the immune cells from injury by free radical production. Supplementation with selenium has increased phagocytic activity and extended the life of macrophages.

Vitamin E

This vitamin may inhibit prostaglandin synthesis that can suppress the immune cells and protects cell membranes as an antioxidant. Supplementation has increased levels of macrophages.

Vitamin A and Caroteniods

Vitamin A supplementation has increased proliferative and cytotoxic responses to T-cells, natural killer (NK) cells and macrophages. It also improves antibody response.

Carotenoids

These antioxidants enhance immune function.

Vitamin C

Vitamin C detoxifies histamine that has an immunosuppressive effect. It acts as an antioxidant and also increases responsiveness of cell-mediated immunity. Given in therapeutic doses (one to four grams/day) at onset of a cold, ascorbic acid reduces the duration of a cold by as much as 48 percent. Vitamin C protects body cells from the oxidizing agent produced by neutrophils. Studies show that during times of infection, even the well-balanced body might not supply sufficient amounts of vitamin C for optimal body function. Vitamin C will also enhance antibiotic therapy.

Fish Oil

The oil found in cold water fish enhances the function of neutrophils and reduces damage to cell membranes.

Garlic

Compounds in garlic have been shown to enhance natural killer (NK) cell activity. Garlic also contains antibacterial agents.

Yogurt

Substances in this fermented food boost gamma interferon.

Pyridoxine (Vitamin B-6)

This B vitamin plays an important role in the production of antibodies. A deficiency of pyridoxine reduces the number of lymphocytes and reduces response of lymphocytes to chemical messengers sent by the T and B lymphocytes.

Sugar

Too much sugar has been shown in vitro to decrease the activity of neutrophils.

DIETARY MODIFICATIONS
TO ENHANCE IMMUNE FUNCTION

1. Eat foods and drink juices that are high in the antioxidant nutrients, vitamin E, beta-carotene, and selenium. Antioxidants will help to protect the membranes of immune cells from being injured by the chemicals they use to battle bacteria with. Sweet peppers, vegetables in the cabbage family, and fruits in the citrus family are excellent sources of vitamin C. Sunflower seeds, almonds, olive oil, and wheat germ are good sources of vitamin E. Orange-fleshed fruits such as papaya and cantaloupe, orange-colored vegetables such as carrots and sweet potatoes, and green leafy vegetables such as spinach and kale are all excellent sources of beta-carotene and the other carotenoids. Wheat germ and whole grains, shellfish such as scallops and shrimp, Brazil nuts and orange juice are good sources of selenium.

2. Include iron-rich foods in your diet. Iron deficiency suppresses the immune system. Foods high in iron include: lean red meat, brewer's yeast, pumpkin seeds and sunflower seeds, raisins, clams, nuts, tofu, and kale.

3. Eat a source of vitamin C with iron-rich foods to enhance absorption of the iron. This antioxidant vitamin also helps to detoxify histamine.

4. Increase your consumption of foods high in zinc and copper. These trace minerals improve immune function. Sources of zinc include: oysters, ginger root, nuts, split peas, whole grains, and chicken. Sources of copper include: oysters, lecithin, nuts, split peas, olive oil, cod liver oil, and whole grains.

5. Eat more cold water fish such as salmon, mackerel, herring, whitefish, lake trout, and halibut. The omega-3 fatty acids in these fish may help to protect the cell membranes of lymphocytes and macrophages from damage.

6. Eat a cup of nonfat yogurt a day. Yogurt made with live cultures of Lactobacillus bulgaricus and Streptococcus thermophilus stimulates the immune cells. Check the label to find the type of bacteria used in making the yogurt.

7. Eat generous amounts of onions, garlic, and leeks. These foods stimulate the immune system.

8. Supplement your diet with brewer's yeast. Sprinkle flakes on your morning cereal or mix powder form with juice drinks. This yeast is very high in vitamin B-6 and iron.

9. Drink alcohol moderately. Alcohol abuse can cause nutritional deficiencies that drain the immune system.

10. Reduce the amount of simple sugars you consume. Excess sugar can reduce the activity of neutrophils.

11. Eat a minimum of five servings of fresh fruits or vegetables each day. Many fruits and vegetables have antibacterial or antiviral action when exposed to microbes. Foods in the cabbage family, apples, grapes, and blueberries all have demonstrated this action.

JUICES FOR
IMMUNE ENHANCEMENT

Asparagus: source of beta-carotene, vitamin E, iron

Blueberries: source of antiviral compounds and iron

Carrots: source of beta-carotene, vitamin E, copper, and zinc

Garlic: source of a natural antibiotic

Grape: source of zinc and antiviral compounds

Kale: source of beta-carotene, vitamin B-6, vitamin C.

Orange: source of vitamin C, the bioflavonoids, and selenium

Papaya: source of beta-carotene, vitamin C

Turnip greens: source of beta-carotene, vitamin B-6, vitamin C

JUICE RECIPES

Immune Booster Shake

Rich in the B vitamins and the immune enhancers found in yogurt and berries.

1 pint strawberries or blueberries
1 tablespoon brewer's yeast powder
1 ripe banana, peeled
½ cup nonfat yogurt

Juice berries and place with the rest of ingredients in a blender. Process until smooth.

Cold Tomato Soup

Rich in protective nutrients, this is the perfect start to a summer meal.

1 tomato
1 clove garlic
½ stalk celery
¼ cup nonfat yogurt

Juice ingredients and stir into yogurt. Pour into bowl and top with croutons.

Iceberry Fizz

An antiviral tonic for your colon.

2 pints blueberries
6 apples
½ lemon
1 inch slice ginger root
sparkling water

See your juicer's instruction for juicing lemons. Remove seeds from apples and juice with ginger. Pour juice into ice cube tray and freeze. Place cubes into blender and crush briefly into a slush. Spoon into glasses and add sparkling water.

Spiced Papaya

Rich in vitamin C and beta-carotene.

2 carrots, tops removed
½ papaya
¼-inch slice ginger root

Prepare papaya according to your juicer's instructions. Juice all ingredients. Pour into glass, garnish with a carrot curl, and serve immediately.

Root Tonic

A combination of two root veggies that are high in essential trace minerals.

½ turnip
2 turnip leaves
5 carrots, tops removed

Juice ingredients.

Sweet Orange Tonic

An excellent source of beta-carotene and potassium.

1 stalk celery, leaves trimmed
½ cantaloupe

Prepare cantaloupe according to your juicer's directions. Juice ingredients. Garnish with a small celery stick.

High-C Citrus Juice

Rich in vitamin C and flavonoids, this juice will help to boost your immune system.

1 orange
½ grapefruit
½ guava
crushed ice

Remove the peel from orange and grapefruit but not the white coat underneath (a source of bioflavonoids). Juice all ingredients. Pour over ice, garnish with an orange slice, and serve immediately.

Vitamin A Special

A drink rich in the carotenes or provitamin A.

4 or 5 carrots, tops removed
2 kale leaves
1 collard leaf

Juice vegetables. Serve immediately.

CHAPTER TEN

Prevention of
Tobacco-Related Diseases

If three full 747 jets crashed each day, every day, would you still fly? Chances are you would be very reluctant. This, however, is how many people die each day of tobacco-related illnesses. Cigarette-associated diseases include: cardiovasular disease (heart disease and stroke), respiratory diseases (chronic obstructive lung disease, emphysema, chronic bronchitis, and sleep disorders), cancers (lung, pharynx, esophagus, bladder, pancreas, and maybe cervical and leukemia), ulcers, problems with pregnancy (mother and child), osteoporosis, diabetes, alcoholism, oral-cavity disease, and accidents. Other problems smokers have are: decreased problem-solving ability, increased depression, increased facial wrinkles, and an increase in sudden death syndrome in infants. You do not even have to smoke to suffer from these disorders. Passive or involuntary smoking occurs when nonsmokers are exposed to smoke in an enclosed environment. The smoke that is not inhaled by the smoker and escapes into the air is actually more toxic than the smoke inhaled directly from the cigarette. Depending upon the circumstances, the level of exposure can reach an equivalent of smoking two cigarettes each day. Children and infants are particularly sensitive to such exposure. If you smoke, stop—if not for yourself then for your family. There are a wide variety of programs designed to help you. If you have tried to stop smoking unsuccessfully in the past, see a counselor for a few sessions to determine what type of program is best suited to your needs. For example, some smokers have a greater physical addiction to nicotine while others have a greater psychological addiction. Some people need one-on-one help, others need group support, or want to go it alone. Don't give up. If you can find the program or combination of programs that fit your needs, you can stop smoking.

HOW DOES TOBACCO CAUSE DISEASE?

When tobacco is burned, it is changed into a complex mixture of gases and solid particles called tar. Over 3,000 components in cigarette smoke have been identified including carbon monoxide, nicotine, nitric acid, the toxic metals arsenic, cadmium, and nickel, and radioactive isotopes. These components can act as initiators of cancer, cocarcinogens, toxins, and genetoxins. Each puff of a cigarette contains ten trillion free radicals in the tar or solid phase and one trillion free radicals in the gas phase. It is these free radicals that are thought to inflict the most damage to human tissue.

NUTRITION AND SMOKING

Not surprisingly, cigarette smoke causes a decrease in the antioxidant nutrients of the body. If you wish to protect yourself or your family from the smoke of others, or if you are a former smoker who wants to repair the damage done by the smoke, the following nutrients are important.

Vitamin C

Smokers have less vitamin C in their plasma and fewer white blood cells than nonsmokers. When this vitamin was given to smokers it improved lung and heart function as well as decreased oxidation of plasma lipoproteins. **Sources of vitamin C include: sweet peppers, citrus fruits, strawberries, cabbage, broccoli, and kale.**

Beta-carotene

Levels of this antioxidant are also lower in smokers. Supplementation of smokers with beta-carotene results in a increased respiratory function and reduced risk of oral cancer. Mothers with high serum levels of beta-carotene who smoke during pregnancy do not have the low-birth weight infants that are common in smoking mothers. **Sources of beta-carotene: carrots, dried apricots, cantaloupe, sweet potatoes, papaya, collard and turnip greens, and kale.**

Vitamin E

Vitamin E levels in the tissue fluid of the lung is lower in smokers. This vitamin is thought to be an important protective nutrient of lung tissue. **Sources of vitamin E: wheat germ oil, sunflower seeds, almonds,** wheat germ, olive oil, peanuts, spinach, oatmeal, asparagus, and salmon.

Vitamin B-6 or Pyridoxine

Smokers have decreased amounts of the biologically active form of this vitamin. **Sources of vitamin B-6 include: brewer's yeast, sunflower seeds, wheat germ, fish (tuna, salmon, trout, halibut, and mackerel), walnuts, beans and lentils, kale, spinach, and turnip greens.**

Folacin

Exposure to cigarette smoke decrease levels of this vitamin in the blood serum and in red blood cells. This leaves the tissue lining of the lungs more susceptible to carcinogens in tobacco. **Sources of folic acid include: brewer's yeast, blackeye peas, wheat germ, beans and lentils, bran and wheat germ, asparagus, spinach, kale, beet and mustard greens, and broccoli.**

Vitamin B-12

The body uses this vitamin to detoxify the cyanide found in smoke. Both tissue and blood levels of B-12 are decreased in smokers. **Sources of B-12 include: shellfish, fish, cheese, eggs, meat, poultry, and milk.** CAUTION: If you do not eat any animal foods or products, you must take a B-12 supplement.

Selenium

This mineral works with vitamin E to prevent free radical damage to cell membranes. Selenium levels have been found to be decreased in smokers. **Sources** of selenium include: whole grains, Brazil nuts, apple cider vinegar, shellfish, red swiss chard, milk, turnips, and garlic.

Zinc

The toxic metal cadmium can concentrate in the placenta of smoking mothers, tying up the zinc the fetus needs for growth. This results in a smaller baby. Sources of zinc include: oysters, ginger root, nuts, split peas, chicken, nonfat dry milk, whole wheat, rye, oats, tuna, haddock, clams, and green peas.

Anutrients and Cancer Blockers and Inhibitors

Smoke contains both promoters and initiators of cancer. For this reason, all of the cancer blockers and suppressors discussed in the chapter on cancer prevention are extremely important in preventing tobacco-related cancers.

JUICES TO HELP PREVENT
TOBACCO-RELATED ILLNESSES

Asparagus: source of folate, and vitamin E
Broccoli: source of vitamin C, folate, and anutrients
Cantaloupe: source of beta-carotene
Carrot: source of beta-carotene, vitamin E, selenium, and zinc
Collards: source of beta-carotene and vitamin C
Ginger: source of zinc
Kale: source of beta-carotene, pyridoxine, vitamin C, folate, and anutrients
Orange: source of selenium, vitamin C, the bio-flavonoids, and anutrients

Spinach: source of vitamin E, zinc, folate, and pyridoxine

Strawberry: source of vitamin C

JUICE RECIPES

Strawberry Fizz

High in vitamin C and selenium.

1 cup strawberries
1 apple, cored
chilled sparkling water

Remove caps from strawberries and juice fruit. Pour into tall glass and fill with sparkling water. Garnish with a whole strawberry.

Berries and Cream

This shake is rich in vitamin C and B-12.

2 cups of strawberries
4 ounces of plain nonfat yogurt

Remove caps from strawberries and juice fruit. Combine juice and yogurt in blender and process until smooth. Pour into glass and garnish with a berry.

The OK Special

The benefits of vegetable juice with a taste like fruit juice. Rich in vitamin C and folate.

3 oranges, peeled
1 kale leaf

Juice ingredients and serve immediately.

Green E Juice

This juice is rich in vitamin E as well as chromium.

1 handful spinach
2 asparagus leaves
1 green pepper
1 carrot, top removed

Juice ingredients. Garnish with a thin asparagus spear and serve immediately.

Four-Veggie Cooler

This drink is rich in pyridoxine, folate, and vitamin C.

tomato juice, frozen into cubes
½ cucumber
2 stalks celery
2 kale leaves

Juice vegetables and pour over tomato cubes. Serve immediately and garnish with a small celery stalk.

Four-Fruit Carotene Snap

This is a drink for those with a sweet tooth.

¼ mango, peeled
¼ papaya, peeled
1 wedge cantaloupe
1 small firm apricot, pitted
½-inch slice ginger root
crushed ice

Follow your juicer's instructions for juicing cantaloupe. Juice fruit and ginger. Pour into tall ice-filled glass.

Simply Orange

An antioxidant powerhouse.

4 or 5 carrots, tops removed
1 orange, peeled

Juice ingredients and garnish with an orange slice.

Carotene Cocktail

This drink contains a blend of the antioxidant carotenoids.

1 tomato
2 carrots
1 collard leaf

Remove top from carrot and juice ingredients. Garnish with a cherry tomato.

ABC Veggie Juice

This combination is high in the antioxidant nutrients.

1 stalk asparagus
2 stalks of broccoli
3 to 5 carrots, tops removed

Remove tops from carrots and juice vegetables. Garnish with a thin asparagus spear and serve immediately.

PART

III

Juicing Through the Life Cycle

CHAPTER ELEVEN

Infants

NEWBORN TO AGE 2

The first two years of life are marked by rapid growth and development. Infants double their birth weight by four months and triple it by the end of their first year. Length increases by 50 percent in one year. Because of this, the foods newborns and infants eat can affect the rest of their lives. For example, infants who develop iron deficiency anemia have a higher risk of having long-term developmental and cognitive problems than babies with normal iron levels.

It is important to remember that infants are not just tiny adults—they have unique nutritional needs because of their age and stage of development. Because of these high energy needs, low-fat high-fiber diets that are recommended for children and adults should not be fed to babies.

IMPORTANT NUTRIENTS
THAT THE INFANT NEEDS

A newborn child will pass through three stages on his way to an adult diet at age two. The diet at each stage must meet the needs of the developing body.

Stage 1: Newborn to 6 Months

The only juice a newborn should receive for the first 5 months is "momjuice" or breastmilk. This is because babies are born with an immature digestive system. The intestine is said to be permeable or "leaky," because large molecules are able to pass through the gut lining and into the bloodstream. The stomach is also immature and unable to produce much acid. When an infant is fed the food it was designed to receive, breastmilk, large molecules and even cells from the mother's breastmilk are able to survive the low acidity of the stomach and be absorbed by the gut. This enhances the immune system and protects the baby from infection. Breastmilk also contains a factor that helps the gut to mature and close so that when solid food is added later, large protein molecules will not be absorbed, possibly causing an allergic reaction. For the first 5 to 6 months, breastmilk or formula (if the mother cannot breast-feed) should be the only food the baby is fed. It contains just the right mix of protein, fat, and energy that the baby's rapidly growing body needs. If other foods or juices are added to the newborn's diet, it can decrease his appetite for milk and decrease his rate of growth. Vegetables offered too early will decrease the amount of iron the baby absorbs from breastmilk and the high levels of nitrites in some vegetables may be turned into cancer-causing nitrosamines in the low-acid stomach of the newborn. Breastmilk contains very little vitamin D and breast-fed infants who are not regularly exposed to the sun may need a supplement at 2 months.

Stage 2: 6 Months to 1 Year

When a baby is about 5 or 6 months old, the iron stores he was born with begin to run out. This is a signal that the baby is ready for solid food. Usually the first food offered is iron-fortified rice cereal that can be moistened with breastmilk or formula. This supplies a baby with needed iron and prevents the infant from developing iron-deficiency anemia. Pureed fruits that contain vitamin C are the next foods offered because this vitamin increases the amount of iron that can be absorbed from a plant food. Always offer juices and foods one at a time to determine if your infant is sensitive or allergic to them. Once the baby has been eating the food or juice for four days with no problems, it can be combined with other foods. Always remove the skins and peels of fruit juiced for babies of this age, strain the juice to remove any foam, and dilute with water.

Some cautions. Be careful not to give too much juice to your baby. It can kill her appetite for breastmilk or formula that should be the main source of nourishment for the first year. Be aware that apple juice will cause diarrhea in some babies so proceed cautiously when you introduce this juice. Never put your baby to bed with a bottle; the sugar in the formula or juice can cause cavities in the baby's lower teeth. For this reason, some pediatricians recommend that infants not be given juice until they can drink it out of a cup.

Stage 3: 1 Year to 2 Years

By now the baby's body has matured. The gut is no longer permeable and stomach acid is at normal strength. The baby is eating a variety of foods and juices and other protein sources besides milk or formula are enjoyed. The young child is now entering a slower phase of growth and his appetite decreases because less food is needed. This makes the 1-year-old much more interested in the process of eating than in the quantity that he is eating. He wants to feed himself and explore the feel and texture of the food inside the mouth and out. Many babies are still breast-feeding but now it's more of a snack and less of a meal. Although the growing baby no longer needs formula, skim or low-fat cow's milk is not yet recommended because the baby still needs fat for growth. Some babies also develop intestinal cramps from low-fat milk. If you choose to give your baby cow's milk, make sure it is whole milk. However, now is an excellent time to introduce soymilk. Although soymilk is naturally rich in protein, it is not a good source of calcium and does not contain vitamin D. Look for the kind that is fortified with calcium and vitamin D and substitute it for milk. Again make sure you feed your baby whole soymilk and not the lower fat or "lite" versions. Older babies love juices and now is the time to instill some good "juicing" habits. Give your toddler two glasses of juice a day. One glass of fruit juice in the morning and one glass of veggie juice at dinner. Let her determine how large a glass she wants.

FOOD ALLERGIES

If either you or your husband have a family history of allergies (food or inhalant), how you feed your infant can have long-lasting consequences. Food allergies occur when protein molecules from a food cross the intestine and are absorbed into the baby's bloodstream, where the body mistakes them for invaders and provokes an immune reaction. Following some simple rules can reduce the chance of your baby developing food allergies and sensitivities and the ear infections they sometimes can cause.

1. Breast-feed your baby for at least one year. Formula feeding with a cow's milk based formula has been associated with increased susceptibility to food allergies and the ear infections, colic, diarrhea, and sleeplessness that cow's milk intolerance can cause.

2. Do not give your baby any wheat, eggs, poultry, or dairy products for the first year. Do not eat any of these products yourself during pregnancy or when you are breast-feeding. These foods are the most likely to cause food allergies and intolerances in susceptible infants and adults.

3. Do not eat any other foods which you or your husband are allergic to during pregnancy and lactation, and do not feed them to your baby during the first year. Food allergies can be inherited.

4. If you cannot breast-feed, I recommend that you substitute a whey hydrolysate formula, such as Carnation's Good Start. Most baby formulas are based on cow's milk and babies who develop allergies to cow's milk formula often develop allergies to soy-based formulas as well. A whey hydrolysate formula contains partially broken down whey proteins that do not stimulate the immune system as cow's milk or soy-milk can.

SUPPLEMENTING THE
BREAST-FEEDING INFANT

Some individuals have recommended feeding fruit and vegetable juices to babies who are less than 6 months old. This practice can cause food allergies and retarded growth because it decreases the amount of milk the baby drinks. But this is not to say that newborns should be deprived of the excellent nutrition they can receive from fresh juice. Newborns should be fed juices in the form of breastmilk. Mom should drink her juices and let nature pass them on to her breast-feeding infant. Think of it as second-hand juicing. Since Mom is now drinking for two, she will need to take baby's tastes into consideration when choosing produce to juice. Drink only small amounts of the stronger tasting juices such as those from the cabbage family (cabbage, broccoli, mustard greens, and Brussels sprouts) and those with levels of oxalates (spinach, beet greens, and Swiss chard). Garlic, in one study, increased the amount of time a group of babies breast-fed. Alcohol on the other hand decreased nursing time.

DIETARY RECOMMENDATIONS FOR THE HEALTHY INFANT

For Children Under 1 Year:

1. Breast-feed your child for at least one year. If that is not possible, breast-feed for as long as possible and then substitute a whey hydrolysate formula. This can be found in your supermarket.

2. Do not let your child have any dairy products until he is at least 1 year old. This will help to prevent allergies and food intolerances.

3. Breastmilk or formula should be the main source of nourishment during your child's first year. Fruits, vegetables, and grains should only supplement the breastmilk or formula, not replace it.

4. Read the section on lactation. Mom should be drinking vitamin-rich juices and, in some cases, taking supplements to pass on to baby.

5. Serve a food or juice rich in vitamin C when you give your child a plant source of iron. Vitamin C increases the absorption of iron from these foods.

6. If either yourself or your husband has a family history of allergies, avoid feeding him the most common allergy-causing foods. These include: wheat, eggs, citrus, milk, and other dairy products.

7. Do not give honey to a child under the age of one year. Honey can contain spores of Clostridium botulinum, the bacteria that causes botulism. Since the immature gut of the infant has fewer defenses than the mature gut of a child or adult, spore-contaminated honey could possibly cause botulism. This ban applies to raw honey as well as cooked and processed honey since Clostridia spores can survive even processing and heating.

8. Do not add salt to a baby's food. Fruits and vegetables contain all the sodium your child needs.

9. Avoid high oxalate foods the first year. These include spinach, beet greens, Swiss chard, and rhubarb. Free oxalates from these foods and juices can bind up the calcium contributed by other foods present in the stomach and reduce the total amount of calcium absorbed from that meal.

10. Let the baby decide when he is full. Never coax him to finish a bottle or clean a plate. If your child will not eat all you give him, decrease serving size.

For Children Over 1 Year

1. During the second year do not give your child any low fat or nonfat dairy products. Use only whole milk, whole yogurt, and whole soymilk. Babies need the fat to grow properly. Babies fed low-fat diets develop "failure to thrive" syndrome.

2. After the baby's first birthday feed her from the table. Buy a simple baby food hand grinder or mash food with your fork. Store-bought baby foods are not necessary. Do not add salt or sugar to food. Foods can be moistened with juice.

3. Never give your child juice in a bottle at night. This causes cavities in your baby's teeth. Fruit juices should be avoided until the child is able to drink them from a cup.

4. Avoid giving your child foods such as hot dogs, nuts, grapes, carrots, and round candies. They can stick in a child's throat and choke her. Thick, sticky foods such as peanut butter can also cause choking by coating the back of the throat.

5. Introduce your child to soyfoods as an alternative to meat and dairy products. Use only fortified soymilk to which vitamin D and calcium are added.

6. Children normally lose interest in food somewhere between 9 and 18 months. The rapid growth of infancy is tapering off and they do not need as much energy as before. Do not be concerned.

JUICES FOR HEALTHY INFANTS

Under 6 Months

Momjuice or breastmilk: source of everything a newborn needs

6 Months to 1 Year

Carrot: source of iron and trace minerals
Orange: source of vitamin C and bioflavonoids
Kale: source of beta-carotene, vitamin C, and iron
Papaya: source of vitamin C
Strawberry: source of vitamin C

For Over 1 Year Add

Apple: source of trace minerals
Cabbage: source of vitamin C
Grapefruit: source of vitamin C
Tomato: source of vitamin C and beta-carotene
Watermelon: source of trace minerals

JUICE RECIPES

Orange Juice

A good first juice that is rich in vitamin C.

1 orange, peeled
water

Juice orange. Pour juice through a strainer and dilute with water. You can store this juice in the refrigerator for up to a day, if you keep the container tightly covered.

Tangerine Juice

Sweeter than orange juice but just as high in vitamin C.

1 tangerine, peeled
water

Juice tangerine. Pour juice through strainer and dilute with water. You can store this juice in the refrigerator for up to a day, if you keep the container tightly covered.

Papaya Surprise

This drink will add a little bit of iron to your child's diet.

¼ papaya
½ kale leaf

Peel papaya and juice with kale leaf. Strain and dilute with a small bit of water.

Apple-Grapefruit Juice

The sweetness of the apple reduces the tartness of the grapefruit. A good source of vitamin C.

½ apple, peeled, cored, and seeded
½ grapefruit, peeled
water

Juice fruit, strain, and dilute with water. You can store this juice in the refrigerator for up to a day, if you keep the container tightly covered.

Strawberry-Orange Treat

A high vitamin C drink.

½ cup strawberries
½ orange, peeled
1 slice of apple, peeled

Remove caps from strawberries and juice fruit. Pour juice through strainer and dilute with water.

First Veggie Juice

A mild-tasting juice suitable for babies over 1 year.

½ tomato
½ stalk celery, leaves trimmed
½ carrot, top removed

Trim leaves off celery and tops off carrot. Juice vegetables and strain.

Carrot/Celery

Rich in minerals and provitamin A.

2 carrots, leaves trimmed
½ stalk celery, top removed
½ small kale leaf

Remove tops from carrots and trim leaves off celery. Juice vegetables and strain.

Garden Patch

A mild-tasting juice that is rich in baby-building minerals.

⅛ head green cabbage
3 carrots, tops removed
1 slice apple, peeled

Juice ingredients and strain. Serve immediately.

CHAPTER TWELVE

Toddlers and Children

AGES 3 TO 9

After the growth spurt of infancy, the child enters a phase of slower growth that will remain constant until the growth spurt at puberty. The infant took only one year to triple his weight. As a toddler it will take him another three years to double his weight. Since fat is no longer needed for rapid growth, a low-fat adult-type diet is recommended. Many health professionals feel that heart disease has its beginnings in childhood with deposits of fatty streaks in the large arteries of the body. This is the age to begin a disease prevention program.

NUTRIENTS NEEDED BY CHILDREN

A child's size may be genetically determined but how much of this size is actually achieved can be a matter decided by good nutrition. Because children are constantly growing new bone, muscle, organ tissue, and blood, they need more nutritious food in proportion to their weight than do adults. Even in this land of plenty, children can be malnourished when they suffer from a prolonged poor appetite, eat a limited number of foods, or eat junk foods with few nutrients. Below are the important nutrients that may be in short supply in children's diets.

Iron

Children between the ages of 1 and 3 are at high risk for iron deficiency. The stores of iron in their bodies have been used up for infant muscle growth and now their diets are typically too low to replenish these stores. Iron-deficiency anemia can cause an increase in the absorption of lead and unfortunately this is the age group most prone to lead poisoning. **Sources of iron include: lean red meat, brewer's yeast, pumpkin seeds and sunflower seeds, raisins and dried prunes, clams, nuts, tofu, kale, wheat germ, and bran.**

Vitamin C

Children often receive less than recommended amounts of vitamin C in their diets. Vitamin C increases the absorption of iron when eaten at the same meal and is also necessary for tissue growth. **Sources include: sweet peppers, kale, collard and turnip greens, broccoli, tomatoes, strawberries, papaya, citrus fruits, mangos, cantaloupes, and cabbage.**

Calcium

Children between 1 and 10 need 800 mg of calcium a day. If a child will not or cannot drink milk, they are at risk for a calcium deficiency. **Sources of calcium include: nonfat dairy products, calcium-fortified soymilk, tofu, corn tortillas, collard leaves, turnip greens, and broccoli.** CAUTION: Although spinach, Swiss chard, and beet greens are often recommended as calcium sources, these greens contain oxalates that bind the calcium, making it unavailable to the body.

Vitamin D

This vitamin is needed for calcium metabolism. Some vitamin D is made when the skin is exposed to sunlight but it is wise to supplement this with pre-formed vitamin D that is present in some foods. If your child drinks milk that is fortified with vitamin D, he is probably not at risk for a deficiency. **Sources of vitamin D include: sardines, salmon, tuna, shrimp, sunflower seeds, liver, eggs, fortified cow's milk, and fortified soymilk.**

Zinc

This trace mineral is necessary for growth and if it is not present in sufficient amounts growth failure, poor appetite, and decreased wound healing can result. Marginal zinc deficiencies have been found in preschool and school-aged children from both low-income and middle-income families. **Sources of zinc include: oysters, ginger root, nuts, split peas, whole grains, and chicken.**

Vitamin B-6

Pyridoxine or vitamin B-6 is needed by the body during periods of growth. **Sources include: brewer's yeast, sunflower seeds, wheat germ, tuna, beans,** salmon, trout, mackerel, brown rice, bananas, halibut, walnuts, hazelnuts, avocados, egg yolks, and kale.

VEGAPHOBIA

A recent survey of children found that 40 percent of those surveyed had not eaten a vegetable other than potatoes or tomato sauce during the last twenty-four hours. Many children steadfastly refuse to eat vegetables. They may not like the strong taste or the texture, or they may just want to be ornery. Forcing a child to eat vegetables is a sure way to make this passing fancy a permanent distaste. Convert the vegaphobic by modeling, not preaching. If you keep eating and enjoying your veggies, sooner or later junior will start to eat and enjoy his as well. While you wait for taste buds to mature, try substituting some of the following foods for vegetables. They will help to fill the nutritional gap left by the absence of vegetables.

Cantaloupe, Mangos, Apricots

If your child will not eat carrots or dark green leafy vegetables, substitute one of these. For example, one cup of cantaloupe contains as much beta-carotene and potassium as one cup of spinach.

Bananas

Celery, Swiss chard, and spinach are rich in potassium and are often recommended to prevent high blood pressure. One banana contains more potassium than any of these veggies, the same amount of pectin as an apple, and more B-6 than any leafy green or root vegetable.

Apples

Beets are known for their detoxifying abilities but the pectin in apples may also be a detoxifier. Studies in Europe suggest that apple pectin may remove lead, mercury, and other toxic-heavy minerals from the body.

Oranges

Peppers, kale, and collard greens are rich sources of vitamin C but so are oranges, papayas, and strawberries. Orange juice is also a good source of folic acid.

Raisins

A ⅔ cup serving of raisins has the same amount of iron as a half cup of parsley and more manganese than a cup of turnip greens or Brussels sprouts and about the same amount of zinc as a cup of carrots.

Ginger

Garlic is famous for its anti–blood clotting abilities. Ginger shares this ability. Since heart disease has its beginnings in childhood, it's never too soon to start thinking heart healthy.

Brewer's yeast

One tablespoon of this yeast powder contains more riboflavin than one cup of mushrooms or collard greens, more pyridoxine than one cup of kale or spinach and the same amount of iron as a cup of kale.

Yogurt

A cup of yogurt contains more magnesium than a cup of collard greens and the same amount of calcium as five cups of broccoli.

Sunflower Seeds

Ounce for ounce, these seeds contain: more B-6 than asparagus or spinach, more potassium and iron than Swiss chard, and more copper than carrots or garlic.

DIETARY RECOMMENDATIONS
FOR HEALTHY CHILDREN

1. Children 2 years and older should follow the guidelines for a healthy heart. To make this easier, stock your shelves with healthy food. Children can't eat junk food if they can't find it. Remove all soda pop, candy, cookies, and other high-fat low-fiber goodies from the house. Make them special foods that are only eaten on special occasions. Remember, children will do what you do, not as you say. Model good eating habits for your child.

2. Substitute juice drinks for soda pop. Some studies have suggested that the phosphates in pop may decrease calcium levels in the body. Many varieties of soda also contain caffeine, a stimulant that may interfere with your child's concentration and sleep.

3. Do not allow your child to skip breakfast. Without breakfast your child will have difficulty concentrating and learning in school. Children who skip breakfast are more likely to overeat later in the day.

4. Snacks are a very important source of nutrition for children in this age group. Just make sure that the snacks you provide are healthy ones. Good snack choices are: unsweetened applesauce (source of pectin), raisins and dried prunes (iron), sunflower seeds (vitamins E, B-6, potassium, and copper), air-popped popcorn (fiber), whole grain dry cereals (fiber), raw fruit and vegetables cut into small, easy to chew pieces (fiber, vitamins, minerals), low-fat yogurt (calcium), and nut butters on whole wheat crackers (protein) or stuffed into celery.

5. Include an iron-rich food and a vitamin C–rich food with every meal to ensure that your child is getting enough iron. Remember, cooking food will reduce its vitamin C content. Cooking acidic foods in an iron pot will increase the iron content. A good example of this is spaghetti sauce. Vitamin C will also counteract the phytate in wheat bread and legumes, making the iron more available for absorption. Always serve your child a vitamin C juice or food along with beans or bread.

6. If high cholesterol runs in your family, substitute soymilk for cow's milk. Children who have familial hypercholesterolemia, an inherited form of high cholesterol, can lower triglyceride and LDL ("bad" cholesterol) levels and raise HDL ("good" cholesterol) levels by substituting soymilk for cow's milk.

7. Children who cannot or will not drink cow's milk should drink calcium and vitamin D–fortified soymilk. Regular soymilk does not contain any vitamin D and only small amounts of calcium. Fortified soymilks come in a variety of flavors designed to appeal to the most finicky child.

8. Supplement your child's diet with wheat germ and brewers yeast. Wheat germ is a good source of fiber, vitamin E, thiamin (B-1), pyridoxine (B-6), folic acid, and selenium. Brewer's yeast is an excellent source of thiamin (B-1), riboflavin (B-2), pyridoxine (B-6), pantothenic acid, biotin, folic acid, niacin, and chromium. Mix equal parts of brewer's yeast flakes with wheat germ, season liberally with cinnamon, and you have a great cereal topping that children love. If your children eat cereal with citrus juice, the topping will also add iron to the diet.

9. Fortify soups, stews, and tomato sauces with green juices. Juices made from low-oxalate green leafy vegetables such as collard greens, turnip greens, and kale will add iron, calcium and other minerals to foods. When added to hearty spicy dishes, they cannot be noticed.

10. Use sweet juices to make natural fruit gelatins and puddings, vegetable juice molded salads, and smoothies.

JUICES FOR HEALTHY CHILDREN

Apple: source of pectin and chromium
Berry: sources of vitamin C
Cantaloupe: source of beta-carotene, vitamin C, and potassium
Carrot: source of beta-carotene, chromium, iron, and zinc
Celery: source of potassium
Ginger: source of zinc and blood thinning factor
Kale: a source of beta-carotene, vitamin C, calcium, iron, and potassium

Orange: source of vitamin C and selenium
Tomato: source of beta-carotene, lycopene, vitamin C, and potassium
Watermelon: source of potassium

JUICE RECIPES

Summertime Punch

This easy-to-make juice will soon be your family's summertime favorite.

2 cups watermelon, cubed
1 orange

Peel oranges and prepare watermelon according to your juicer's instructions. Pour over crushed ice, shake, and strain juice into glasses.

Fizzy C Cooler

Vitamin C that tickles your nose.

1 papaya
¼-inch slice ginger root
chilled sparkling water
ice cubes

Peel papaya and juice with ginger. Pour into glass over ice and add sparkling water.

Cherry Surprise

A healthy frozen treat with a surprise in the middle.

1 cup cherry or other red berry juice
1 cup apple juice
six 2-inch banana slices
six 5-oz. paper cups
6 wooden sticks

Mix juices together. Push wooden sticks through banana slices and place one in each cup. Pour about 2½ ounces of juice into each cup and freeze.

Frozen Strawberry Yogurt

Vitamin C and calcium in one treat.

12 ounces strawberry juice
1½ cups nonfat plain yogurt
5 oz. paper cups
wooden sticks

Combine juice and yogurt and fill paper cups ⅔ full with mixture. Add sticks and freeze.

Sweet Orange Tonic

An excellent source of beta-carotene and potassium.

1 stalk celery, leaves trimmed
½ cantaloupe

Prepare cantaloupe according to your juicer's directions. Juice ingredients. Garnish with a small celery stick.

Strawberry Gello

Superior in every way to the artificially flavored desserts.

1 cup of berry juice (strawberry, blueberry, loganberry)
1 cup red grape juice
1 package unflavored gelatin

Mix 1 cup berry juice with 1 cup grape juice. Pour ½ cup juice mixture into a small saucepan and sprinkle gelatin on top. Heat gently while stirring, until gelatin dissolves. Remove from heat and add remaining cold juice. Pour into dishes and chill until set.

Salad Gel

Let your kids eat their vegetable juice. Rich in vitamin C and carotenes.

1¼ cup tomato juice
½ cup celery juice
¼ cup red sweet pepper juice
1 envelope unflavored gelatin

Mix juices and pour ½ cup into small saucepan. Sprinkle gelatin on top of juice, heat gently, and stir until gelatin dissolves. Add remaining juice and pour into molds or dishes. Garnish with grated carrot.

Chocolate and Strawberries

A calcium and vitamin C rich drink tempting enough for an adult.

¾ cup cocoa flavored calcium-fortified soymilk
¼ cup strawberry juice

Mix ingredients and garnish with a strawberry.

CHAPTER THIRTEEN

Teens and Young Adults

AGES 10 TO 29

At this stage of the life cycle, the rate of growth again increases. At puberty, the adolescent bursts into adulthood with what is known as the growth spurt. For girls this begins shortly after 10 years of age and peaks at about 12, with the weight growth spurt beginning about 6 months later. For boys the growth height spurt begins at about 12 and peaks at 14. Thus for girls the period of greatest nutritional need is between 10 and 13 years of age and for boys between 12 and 15 years. Girls begin menstruation after the weight spurt when they reach about 103 pounds and fat stores have doubled from the 10 percent fat of a child to the 20 percent of womanhood. A body composition of at least 22 percent fat is necessary to maintain regular ovulation. For boys, sexual development starts at the beginning of the growth spurt and continues for two and a half to three years.

During adolescence and young adulthood, the male

body appears to be very forgiving to dietary indiscretions. Young males can often eat large quantities of food, including fat, and still be fit, trim and muscular. Externally they appear to be healthy, but internally arteries are silently clogging. Young women, on the other hand, often begin what amounts to be a life-long deprivation diet in an effect to achieve impossible weight goals. The amount of calories they consume is often too low to provide proper levels of nutrients.

Both men and women reach full growth between the ages of 18 and 20 years but bone growth continues to increase until the age of 25. Mature women have twice as much fatty tissue as men and two thirds as much muscle tissue.

NUTRIENTS NEEDED BY ADOLESCENTS DURING RAPID GROWTH

During puberty there is a rapid enlargement of the major organs, muscles, and bones. Sexual maturity complicates matters with its changes in psychological and physiological functioning. Although all vitamins and minerals are important for proper growth, today's teens' diets lack the following nutrients:

MINERALS

During the adolescent growth spurt, almost twice the amount of calcium, iron, and zinc is added to the adolescent body than during the preceding childhood years.

Calcium

This mineral is needed for the growing skeleton and

for the proper functioning of the muscles. Good sources of calcium include: nonfat dairy products, calcium-fortified soymilk, tofu, corn tortillas, collard leaves, turnip greens, and broccoli. CAUTION: Although spinach, Swiss chard and beet greens are often recommended as calcium sources, these greens contain oxalates that bind the calcium, making it unavailable to the body. This is especially true for their juices, which may react with other calcium sources in your stomach to reduce the total amount of calcium you absorb from the meal.

Iron

This mineral is an important part of lean muscle tissue and young men need extra amounts of it during rapid growth. Although young women do not gain as much muscle tissue as young men, they will lose more iron because of the menstrual cycle. Sources of iron include: lean red meat, brewer's yeast, pumpkin seeds and sunflower seeds, raisins and dried prunes, clams, nuts, tofu, kale, wheat germ, and bran. Cooking acidic foods in an iron pot will increase the iron content of the foods cooked in them. A good example of this is spaghetti sauce. Vitamin C will counteract the phytate in wheat bread and legumes, making the iron more available for absorption, so always have a vitamin C juice or food along with beans or bread.

Zinc

This trace mineral is essential for growth. During the growth spurt the body becomes more efficient at absorbing this mineral. Sources of zinc include: oysters, ginger root, nuts, split peas, whole grains, and chicken.

VITAMINS

Vitamin A

This fat-soluble vitamin is needed for tissue development and growth. Low levels of vitamin A were found in 10 to 40 percent of the teenagers studied in the Ten State Nutrition Study. Sources of vitamin A include: liver, whitefish, swordfish, eggs, chicken, and cod liver oil. Sources of provitamin A (which is converted to vitamin A by the body) include: carrots, dried apricots, sweet potatoes, butternut squash, collards, and kale.

Vitamin D

Vitamin D is necessary for proper bone metabolism and is especially needed during periods of rapid growth. Sources of vitamin D include: sardines, salmon, tuna, shrimp, sunflower seeds, liver, eggs, fortified cow's milk, and fortified soymilk.

Vitamin C

Increased amounts of ascorbic acid is needed during periods of rapid growth, inhaling smoke (yours and others), and taking oral contraceptives. Vitamin C will also increase the amount of iron that is absorbed from meals that contain nonheme (nonanimal) sources of iron. Sources of vitamin C include: sweet peppers, kale, collard and turnip greens, broccoli, strawberries, papaya, citrus fruits, mangos, cantaloupes, and cabbage.

Folacin (Folic Acid)

This B vitamin is needed for RNA synthesis and levels have been found to be especially low in pregnant teens. Sources of folacin include: brewer's yeast, wheat germ, beans, asparagus, spinach, kale, beet and mustard greens, broccoli, whole wheat, cabbage, oatmeal, and split peas.

Pyridoxine (B-6)

Another B vitamin that is often low in women who take oral contraceptives. Sources include: brewer's yeast, sunflower seeds, wheat germ, tuna, beans, salmon, trout, mackerel, brown rice, bananas, halibut, walnuts, hazelnuts, avocados, egg yolks, and kale.

Vitamin B-12

Vitamin B-12 is involved in protein, fat, and carbohydrate metabolism. Sources include: shellfish, fish, eggs, cheese, and milk. CAUTION: Vegetarians who eat no animal products must supplement this vitamin.

Niacin, Riboflavin, and Thiamin

These B vitamins are involved in energy metabolism and are needed in extra amounts during adolescence. Sources of niacin include: brewer's yeast, wheat bran, peanuts, light meat from poultry, fish, sunflower and sesame seeds, pine nuts, and brown rice. Sources of riboflavin include: brewer's yeast, almonds, wheat germ, wild rice, mushrooms, millet, mackerel, soybeans, eggs, and split peas. Sources of thiamin include: brewer's yeast, wheat germ, nuts, beans, whole grains, split peas, mung beans, and lentils.

NUTRITION FOR YOUNG WOMEN ON ORAL CONTRACEPTIVES

Oral contraceptives (OCs) are made of synthetic hormone preparations. Most OCs today are combinations of estrogen and progestogens that are prescribed in dosages that are much less than the original pills and they also have fewer nutritional side effects. Only two vitamins are at risk for deficiency: pyridoxine (B-6) and folacin (folic acid). Sources of these vitamins are listed above.

PREPARING FOR CONCEPTION AND PREGNANCY

During young adulthood many couples will decide to start a family. But before you start shopping for baby furniture, evaluate your own internal crib. Are you in good enough nutritional shape to nourish a child optimally? Diet is one of the most important factors influencing the outcome of pregnancy. The growing child has no source of nutrients other than the mother's food and nutrient stores. How adequate these nutrient stores are depends upon the foods she eats before she becomes pregnant. For example, a vitamin deficiency in the period before conception, especially a folacin deficiency, is linked to birth defects involving the neural tube. Let us also not forget Dad. Women are born with their eggs already formed, but men are constantly making new supplies of sperm and it only makes sense that a man's nutritional and physical health affects the quality of the sperm he produces.

JUICING FOR GOOD HEALTH

PREPREGNANCY NEEDS OF WOMEN

Folacin, Vitamin C, and Riboflavin

Women who have given birth to a child with a malformation of the neural tube have been found to be lacking in these vitamins.

Folacin and Pyridoxine (B-6)

These two B complex vitamins are lost in women who have taken contraceptives. If you have taken OCs be sure to supplement your diet with brewer's yeast to replenish all the B vitamins.

Chromium

Low levels of this trace mineral may be associated with glucose intolerance during pregnancy.

Iron

Since the baby has to store six months' worth of iron in his liver, the prospective mother needs to have large iron stores in her liver before conception.

Zinc

This trace mineral is needed very early in pregnancy. By the time a woman realizes she is pregnant, the period when zinc levels are most important has passed.

OTHER LIFESTYLE FACTORS

Caffeine in coffee and soft drinks

Caffeine in these beverages (but not in tea) was linked to decreased fertility in one study. As little as one caffeinated soft drink was enough to decrease fertility by 50 percent!

Underweight

Chronic dieting can lead to an absence of menstruation and ovulation. If you want to conceive, concentrate on eating healthy, not on counting calories.

Drugs and Alcohol

Moderately heavy drinkers experience a higher rate of miscarriage, *abruptio placentae,* and low-birthweight delivery in addition to the risk of fetal alcohol syndrome. Since researchers do not yet know how much alcohol is too much alcohol, parents who want to produce a child with optimal health should not drink.

Tobacco Use

Cigarette smoke contains the heavy metal cadmium. This mineral may build up in the placenta, interfering with zinc absorption, which then causes reduced growth in the unborn baby. If you are planning a pregnancy and are constantly exposed to cigarette smoke, ask your physician or midwife about taking a zinc supplement. Cigarette smokers also have higher lead and mercury levels than nonsmokers but how this affects the fetus is unknown. Read the chapter on tobacco-related diseases for more information.

FERTILITY AND MEN

Mounting evidence suggests that environmental factors can affect the quality of sperm. For example, the children of firefighters are more likely to have congenital heart defects, possibly because of their fathers' exposure to toxic fumes.

Copper

This trace element may be involved in the maturation of sperm and is part of an enzyme that neutralizes free radicals that may cause infertility.

High Fat Diets

A typical Western diet that is high in fat may be linked to low testosterone levels.

Alcohol

Some evidence suggests a relationship between the paternal use of alcohol and the size of his offspring. Any man who wants to become a father should prepare his body for fatherhood as well.

DIETARY RECOMMENDATIONS
FOR HEALTHY YOUNG MEN AND WOMEN

1. Both men and women should follow a heart healthy diet. Fatty streaks present in the arteries of children turn into fibrous plaques in the arteries of teens. Now is the time to prevent these plaques from growing and clogging arteries. A diet and exercise program that will prevent heart disease in men will also help prevent osteoporosis in women.

2. Both men and women should drink three glasses of calcium fortified soymilk or nonfat cow's milk each day. This will help to increase bone mass and protect you from developing osteoporosis later in life.

3. If you smoke occasionally or inhale the smoke of others, eat foods rich in antioxidant nutrients. This includes citrus fruits and yellow and green fruits and vegetables.

4. If you drink occasionally, replace the nutrients lost when your body processes the alcohol. The metabolism of alcohol requires the B vitamins and magnesium. Sources of B vitamins and magnesium are: brewer's yeast, wheat germ, sunflower seeds, and nuts.

5. No matter how busy you are, always eat breakfast. At least one third of your day's calories should be eaten in the morning. Breakfast refuels your brain after the night's fast and will increase your ability to concentrate at work or school.

6. If you want to drop to a smaller clothes size:

- Concentrate on decreasing the fat in your diet, not the calories.
- Eat more raw fruits and vegetables, at least seven servings a day.
- Eat less fat, and no fried food or fatty foods.
- Do not use sugar.
- Limit the amount of fruit juice you drink. Drink more vegetable juice.

- Eliminate alcoholic beverages.
- Exercise, exercise, exercise. A daily walk is a good way to start an exercise program.
- Always eat breakfast.

7. If you want to gain a clothes size:

- Concentrate on increasing complex carbohydrates, not fats.
- Increase the amount of starchy fruits and vegetables you eat including bananas, potatoes, sweet potatoes, and corn.
- Eat more whole grains and legumes.
- Join an exercise program with weight training to increase muscle size.
- Be aware of food supplements that claim to increase muscle mass; these products do not work. Equally ineffective are protein powders.

8. If you are preparing to become pregnant:

- Avoid toxins in your environment.
- Do not drink or use recreational drugs of any kind.
- Follow the disease prevention diet in Chapter 14.
- The prospective mother should eat a diet high in iron and calcium and supplement her diet with a chromium enriched brewer's yeast supplement.
- Limit the amount of caffeine-containing drinks you consume to two a day. This includes caffeine-containing soft drinks and coffee.
- Do not smoke or inhale the smoke of others.

JUICES FOR HEALTHY YOUNG ADULTS

Apple: source of chromium
Broccoli: source of riboflavin, pantothenic acid, folacin, calcium, magnesium, and iron
Cabbage: source of vitamin C and zinc
Carrot: source of iron, copper, chromium, and zinc
Collards: source of riboflavin, calcium, and magnesium
Ginger root: source of copper and zinc
Green pepper: source of vitamin C and chromium
Kale: source of riboflavin, pyridoxine, folacin, and vitamin C
Orange: source of vitamin C and selenium
Papaya: source of vitamin C and copper
Romaine: source of calcium
Strawberry: source of vitamin C and iron
Turnip greens: source of pyridoxine (B-6) and calcium

JUICE RECIPES

Weight Booster

Drink this shake each day and it will help to maximize your weight without clogging your arteries.

1 orange, peeled
1 papaya, peeled
1 ripe banana, peeled
1 tablespoon brewer's yeast powder

Juice orange and papaya. Combine juice with banana and yeast powder in blender and process until smooth. Garnish with an orange slice.

Citrus Sparkler

A not-too-sweet party drink.

1 grapefruit, peeled
½ orange, peeled
½ slice ginger root
chilled sparkling water

Juice ingredients, pour over ice, and add sparkling water.

Flower Power Cocktail

Rich in antioxidants, down one of these when you find yourself in a smoky room.

1 stalk broccoli
1 stalk cauliflower
½ green pepper
1 tomato

Juice vegetables, garnish with a slice of pepper, and serve immediately.

Berrymint Cooler

A cool way to get your vitamin C.

strawberry juice, frozen into cubes
2 oranges, peeled
handful fresh mint
1 apple, seeded

Juice fruit and mint. Pour into tall glass, add strawberry cubes, and garnish with a mint sprig.

Citrus Zinger

A good drink to get you going in the morning without caffeine.

one 2-inch slice of pineapple
¼ grapefruit, peeled
½ orange, peeled
½ inch slice ginger root
chilled sparkling water

Prepare pineapple according to your juicer's directions. Juice ingredients. Pour into a tall glass and add sparkling water. This juice can be prepared in the evening and stored in the refrigerator overnight. Add sparkling water just before serving.

Red Hot Tomato Cooler

Love spicy food? This is a hot way to get your vitamin C.

3 tomatoes
1 collard leaf
¼-inch slice of hot red pepper

Juice ingredients, being careful not to touch the pepper juice.

Turnip Tonic

A surprisingly sweet drink rich in cancer preventative agents.

½ medium rutabaga
½ turnip, top removed
2 carrots, tops removed

Juice ingredients.

Georgie B. Special

A broccoli drink even a President could love.

1 broccoli spear
3 apples, seeded
½ firm pear, seeded

Juice ingredients and serve immediately.

Smokers' Special

This drink will aid in replenishing the antioxidants lost to cigarette smoke while you join a stop-smoking program. It is also rich in cancer-protective agents.

3 spears asparagus
1 handful spinach leaves
3 to 4 carrots, tops removed

Juice ingredients and serve immediately.

CHAPTER FOURTEEN

Mature Adults

AGES 30 TO 60

We spend the largest portion of our life in this stage of the life cycle, which spans from the early 30s to the mid-60s. This is the time in our lives when we either reap the benefits of good lifestyle choices or suffer the consequences of poor lifestyle choices. It is also time to prepare for the senior years. Establishing good nutrition habits now will help to maximize your health later by preventing or delaying chronic diseases.

During the mature years, body composition again changes. In men, the amount of lean tissue decreases and is replaced by fatty tissue. This is why many men find their waist size growing while their weight stays the same. The decrease in muscle tissue also means that the body will now need less energy (calories) to fuel itself.

MENOPAUSE AND NUTRITION

Menopause is the result of decreasing estrogen production by the ovaries. As estrogen levels decline, menstrual periods become lighter and irregular and then stop altogether. The ovaries will still continue to produce androgens that are responsible for muscular strength and sex drive, but the loss of estrogen can mean hot flashes, vaginal dryness, and osteoporosis for some women. Here are some guidelines that may help reduce symptoms.

1. Exercise, exercise, exercise. It will help to build bone and may relieve hot flashes in some women. If you are not used to exercise, start by walking a half hour each day.

2. Reduce alcohol and caffeine. These drinks can aggravate hot flashes in some women.

3. If your doctor recommends calcium supplementation to prevent osteoporosis, remember that calcium is only one part of the bone matrix. Wash down your pills with plenty of juice to provide trace minerals and vitamin cofactors that will help build bone mass.

4. Increase the amount of soy products in your diet. These foods contain substances called phytoestrogens. Phytoestrogens gently supplement the natural estrogens in your body without increasing the risk of breast cancer. When soyflour was fed to postmenopausal women, vaginal dryness decreased after eight weeks. Soy products include: tofu, soybeans, soymilk, tempeh, and soyflour. Other sources of phytoestrogens include: asparagus, beets, Brussels sprouts, cauliflower, loose-leaf lettuce, okra, and apricots.

5. Follow a heart healthy diet. The loss of estrogen's protective effect means that the postmenopausal woman runs the same risk of heart disease as a man.

6. If your doctor recommends estrogen replacement therapy, increase the amount of vegetables you eat from the cruciferous family. An unidentified component of these foods may help to detoxify estrogen in the body, preventing women with a family history of hormone-dependent breast cancer from developing this disease. Cruciferous vegetables include: cabbage, broccoli, cauliflower, Brussels sprouts, mustard greens, and kale.

NUTRITION AND THE SKIN

One of the most distressing signs of middle age is the deepening of wrinkles. Wrinkles are the result of changes in the deeper layers of the skin that are manifested on the surface of the skin. While there is no way to permanently erase wrinkles, certain dietary and lifestyle changes can help to minimize them.

1. What is the difference between a smooth plump grape and a dry wrinkled raisin? Just a little water. Drink eight to ten glasses of water a day in the form of vegetable juices, diluted fruit juices, herbal teas, or plain water. Water helps the skin resist the forces that cause it to buckle and fold.

2. Silicone is part of collagen and elastin, proteins that are essential for the formation of connective tissue. The highest silicon concentrations are found in the skin and these concentrations decrease with age. Sources of silicone include: beer, unrefined grains, and root vegetables.

3. Zinc is a busy mineral involved with over ninety enzymes in the body including those responsible for cell division and collagen synthesis in the skin. A deficiency in zinc results in slow wound healing. Sources of zinc include: fresh oysters, pumpkin seeds, ginger root, nuts, legumes, beef liver, nonfat milk and

yogurt, egg yolk, whole wheat, leafy and root vegetables.

4. Vitamin C is an antioxidant that protects the delicate membranes of skin cells from attack by free radicals. Vitamin C is also necessary to build collagen and support the immune system. The bioflavonoids work with vitamin C to help strengthen capillary walls. Sources of vitamin C include: raw leafy vegetables, tomatoes, peppers, broccoli, Brussels sprouts, strawberries, cabbage, citrus fruits, and cantaloupe.

5. Don't smoke. Smoking causes deep crevasses in the skin.

6. Reduce the amount of tea and coffee you drink. These beverages have a diuretic effect that causes your skin to lose precious water.

7. Always wear a sunscreen with a sun protection factor (SPF) of at least fifteen. Most of the lines and wrinkles on the face are due to exposure to the ultraviolet rays of the sun. A good sunscreen can prevent not only wrinkling but skin cancer and damage to the immune system. Remember, a tan is not a sign of health, it is a signal that the skin has been damaged.

DIETARY RECOMMENDATIONS TO HELP PREVENT PREMATURE DEATH

1. Replace all vegetable oils and animal fats with olive oil. Use canola or high oleic safflower oil occasionally for foods that need a lighter tasting oil. The monounsaturated fats in these oils will help to prevent heart disease.

2. Replace half of the milk you drink with low-fat calcium-fortified soymilk and eliminate all dairy products with fat. Consume only skim milk, nonfat cheeses, and nonfat yogurt. Whole milk dairy products are sources of saturated fat that may cause your cholesterol and blood pressure to climb. Soymilk contains cancer-fighting anutrients, cholesterol lowering protein, and phytosterols that can supplement estrogen.

3. Eat only whole grain foods such as whole grain breads, whole grain cereals, and brown rice. The fiber and phytate in these foods may help prevent colon cancer.

4. Eat at least five servings of vegetables each day. This should include: one serving of orange or yellow vegetables, two servings of calcium-rich leafy green vegetables, and one serving from the cabbage family. Raw fruits and vegetables are a treasure chest of preventative chemicals for all the major killer diseases.

5. Eat at least two servings of whole raw fruit each day, including one citrus. Eat at least six different kinds of fruit each week.

6. Decrease the amount of animal flesh you eat. Eat no more one serving of low-fat red meat each week. Eat no more than one serving of animal flesh each day. At least three times a week, this animal flesh should be a cold water fish. All poultry should be skinless and trimmed of visible fat. These modifications will change the types and amount of fat you consume each week, decreasing your chances of developing cancer, heart disease, stroke, hypertension, and diabetes.

7. Increase the amount of beans and lentils in your diet. This includes at least one form of soyfood each day in the form of low-fat soymilk, tofu, tempeh, soybeans, or soyflour and one cup of cooked beans or lentils each day. This will increase the amount of cholesterol-absorbing fiber in your diet as well as reduce your chances of colon cancer.

8. Cook food properly. Fish and pork should not be cooked in the microwave. The internal temperatures of pork and fish do not reach a high enough temperature to kill disease-causing parasites. Animal flesh should not be grilled over high heat or over an open flame. This can lead to the formation of cancer-causing polycyclic hydrocarbons. Eat only one serving of fried food a month (this includes french fries, potato chips, corn chips, etc.) and air-pop popcorn to reduce fat intake.

9. Drink no more than two cups or glasses of a caffeine-containing beverage each day. High coffee consumption has been linked to high blood pressure, heart disease, and stomach pain and caffeine may increase hot flashes in menopausal women. Caffeine is also a diuretic, a substance that causes water loss, and too much of it can lead to dehydration. Beverages that contain caffeine include: coffee, tea, colas, and some other soft drinks.

10. Reduce your salt intake. Do not cook vegetables in salt and ban the salt shaker from the table. Substitute fresh lemon juice and herb mixtures. A high salt intake has been linked to high blood pressure, osteoporosis, and stroke.

11. Drink eight to ten glasses of water each day. Water helps your kidneys to excrete toxins and your skin to hydrate, "plumping up" those wrinkles on your face.

12. Decrease the amount of sugar you eat. As the body matures, it produces less insulin that is needed for the cells to utilize sugar. A high sugar intake may also depress the immune system.

13. Drink at least two glasses of vegetable juice and one glass of diluted fruit juice each day. Fresh juice will supply your body with extra vitamins, minerals, and anutrients to protect it from today's hazardous environment.

JUICES FOR A PRODUCTIVE MIDDLE AGE

Apple: source of antiviral compounds and chromium

Broccoli: source of antioxidants, cancer blocking and suppressive agents, phytosterols, calcium, magnesium, and folacin

Cabbage: source of antioxidants, cancer blocking and suppressive agents, phytosterols, calcium, magnesium, and folacin

Carrot: source of carotenes, copper, zinc, and silicone

Garlic: source of cancer blocking and suppressive agents, compounds that lower blood pressure and cholesterol, and compounds that thin the blood

Ginger: source of zinc, copper, and blood thinners

Grapefruit: source of vitamin C, bioflavonoids, and pectin

Lemon: source of vitamin C, the bioflavonoids, and also a good salt substitute

JUICE RECIPES

Vitamin A Special

A drink rich in the carotenes or provitamin A.

4 or 5 carrots, tops removed
2 kale leaves
1 collard leaf

Juice vegetables. Serve immediately.

Vitamin B Special

The brewer's yeast gives this almost every B vitamin.

3 oranges, peeled
1 banana, peeled
1 tablespoon brewer's yeast

Combine orange juice with banana and yeast in a blender. Process until smooth.

Menapausal Firequencher

High in phytoestrogens, this drink may put out your hot flashes. Try it for a quick breakfast.

4 to 6 apricots
2 cups loose leaf lettuce
1 ripe banana, peeled
2 tablespoons soy protein

Remove stones from apricots and juice them with the lettuce. Add juice, banana, and soy to blender and process until smooth.

Wrinkle Reducer

This is a low calorie high antioxidant drink that will help plump up your wrinkles while it helps to nourish your skin.

2 kiwi fruits, peeled
1 orange, peeled
sparkling water

Juice fruit. Pour over ice and fill glass to the top with chilled sparkling water.

The Estrogen Detoxifier

Compounds in this juice may aid in detoxifying estrogen, thereby decreasing the chance of developing hormone-dependent breast cancer.

¼ head of cabbage
1 broccoli stalk
1 kale leaf
2 carrots, tops removed

Juice ingredients. Serve immediately.

Chromium Cocktail

High in chromium and low in sugar, this drink will help your body use glucose more efficiently.

1 green pepper
3 green apples, seeded

Juice ingredients. Serve immediately.

Root Tonic

A tasty way to get the trace minerals present in root vegetables.

4 carrots, tops removed
½ medium rutabaga
1 small turnip

Juice ingredients. Serve immediately.

Kiwi Tea

Spicy and full of vitamin C, try this drink instead of coffee. The green tea contains epigallacatechin gallate, an anutrient that is a suppressive agent (prevents cancer promotion). It is particularly effective against smoke-induced lung cancer.

1 kiwi fruit, peeled
¼-inch slice ginger root
green tea bag

Juice kiwi with ginger. Brew six ounces of tea and combine with juices. Serve hot.

CHAPTER FIFTEEN

Seniors

OVER 60

The senior cycle of life can be divided into two broad groups, the "young" seniors and the "old" seniors. Although young seniors are healthy and active, they need to learn how to adapt their diets to their bodies' changing needs so they can stay healthy and delay the onset of chronic disease.

Old seniors are frail and suffer from chronic diseases. They require assistance in preparing meals and making juices and often are on multiple medications that may cause them to lose their appetites. The positive effects of good nutrition for this age group cannot be underestimated. Even in healthy older adults with no signs of clinical nutrient deficiencies, research has found an association between nutritional status and cognitive function. Because seniors eat smaller amounts of food, they need to eat foods with a high nutritional density. Juices and food supplements can provide the concentrated nutrients this group needs.

CHANGES IN THE BODY
DURING THE SENIOR YEARS

After the body has reached maturity, the rate at which bodily processes occur begins to decrease. The loss of cells becomes greater than the regeneration of cells. The following changes occur in the senior body and must be compensated for in the diet.

1. The number of taste buds on the tongue decreases. Foods previously enjoyed now become "tasteless." This can lead to loss of appetite and poor nutrition.

2. The salivary glands reduce the amount of saliva they produce. This results in a chronically dry mouth that makes chewing and swallowing difficult. Avoid giving seniors dry foods such as crackers and bread. Moisten foods with juices or milk to make them easier to swallow. Saliva substitutes are also available without prescription at your pharmacy.

3. Bone loss in the upper and lower jaws can result in tooth loss and ill-fitting dentures. This makes chewing difficult or painful and can lead to poor nutrition. If a sore mouth is the problem, serve only soft foods such as mashed potatoes and soft fruits, finely chopped foods such as cooked ground meat, and grated foods such as raw vegetables. All seniors with dentures should see their dentist once a year to have their plates adjusted.

4. The stomach decreases the amount of hydrochloric acid it secretes. This can cause malabsorption of some nutrients such as calcium, iron, and vitamin B-12 and it may be necessary to take an acid supplement with meals. Ask your physician about prescribing one.

5. Bile secretion is decreased, which makes fat absorption less efficient. Avoid high-fat foods such as

whole milk, cheese, ice cream, pies, salad dressing, oils, butter, margarine, fried foods, fatty meat, and poultry skin. In severe cases of malabsorption, it may be necessary to supplement the diet with *medium chain triglycerides (MCTs)*, a type of fat that is easily absorbed. MCT supplements are available without prescription at your pharmacy.

6. The muscle movements of the intestines decrease. This can cause the movement of food through the digestive tract to slow, resulting in constipation. Increasing the amount of fluid and the amount of fiber in the diet will help relieve this. If your doctor recommends a fiber laxative, purchase one that contains at least two different sources of fiber and then mix it with fresh juice.

7. The pancreas secretes less insulin, resulting in high blood sugar levels after meals high in simple sugars. Cells also become resistant to insulin. This can be avoided by eating complex carbohydrates (breads, potatoes, pasta) and cutting down on simple sugars (fruit juices, cakes, candies). Read the chapter on noninsulin dependent diabetes for more information.

8. Appetite decrease. Very often your medication can cause a loss of appetite. Be sure to report this to your doctor. Yet even when you aren't hungry, drinks and smoothies can be enjoyed. And juices combined with proteins are an effective way of providing nutrition to undernourished seniors.

NUTRIENTS NEEDED BY SENIORS

Sources of each nutrient are listed but because of reduced absorption, it may be necessary to supplement some of these nutrients in pill form.

Protein

Infections, decreased gastrointestinal function, and changes in metabolism caused by chronic disease can lessen protein's benefit on the body. Signs of a protein deficiency include: edema, itchy skin, chronic eczema, fatigue, muscle weakness, and tissue wastage. **Good sources of protein include: low-fat cow's milk, soymilk, soyfoods such as tofu, lean-red meat, skinless poultry, beans, split peas and lentils when eaten with whole grains such as rice and bread.**

Vitamin B-12

This vitamin is not well absorbed by seniors. Ask your physician about B-12 injections. **Sources of B-12 include: shellfish, fish, egg yolks, and lean beef. Vegetarians should supplement this vitamin.**

Folacin

A deficiency of this B vitamin has been reported to cause degeneration of the intestinal lining, which can further reduce nutrient absorption. **Sources of folacin include: brewer's yeast, soy flour and beans, wheat germ, beans, lentils, walnuts and filbert nuts, peanuts, and split peas.**

Thiamin (Vitamin B-1)

A deficiency in this B vitamin can cause loss of appetite, irritability, fatigue, depression, sleep disorders, and weight loss. **Sources of thiamin include: brewer's yeast, wheat germ, nuts, beans, whole grains, split peas, mung beans, and lentils.** Antacids can interfere with the absorption of this vitamin.

Pyridoxine (Vitamin B-6)

The elderly may need more of this vitamin than is currently recommended. A deficiency reduces immune function and can lead to depression. **Sources of pyridoxine include: brewer's yeast, sunflower seeds, wheat germ, fish, beans, nuts, bananas, and whole wheat flour.**

Vitamin D

Studies indicate that seniors often have low levels of this fat-soluble vitamin. This is due to a decrease of dietary sources of vitamin D and decreased absorption, decreased ability to transform vitamin D into its active form. A lack of vitamin D can result in softening of the bones (osteomalcia), bone pain, and muscle weakness. **Sources of vitamin D include: canned sardines, salmon, fresh tuna, shrimp, sunflower seeds, eggs, mushrooms, fortified cow's milk, and fortified soymilk.**

Calcium

Many of the factors that determine how well calcium is absorbed and used are affected by the aging of the body. Intestinal absorption of calcium decreases and the hormone levels that regulate bone formation decrease. **Sources of calcium include: low-fat cow's milk, calcium fortified soymilk, collard leaves, kale, turnip greens, tofu, nonfat yogurt, goat's milk, broccoli, and romaine lettuce.**

Chromium

Low levels of chromium may be related to glucose resistance and some types of heart disease. Levels of this nutrient decrease with age. **Sources of chromium include: apples, barley and other whole grains, brewer's yeast, and acidic foods that have been in contact with stainless steel.**

Copper

Copper levels are often low in persons who have liver disease, rheumatoid arthritis, atherosclerosis, high blood pressure, cancer or an infection. **Sources of copper include: oysters, lecithin, nuts, split peas, olive oil, cod liver oil, and whole grains.**

Iron

Iron requirements are lowest in old age. However, iron from plant sources needs an acidic environment to be absorbed and low levels of stomach acid (achlorhydria) are common in the elderly. **Sources of iron include: lean red meat, brewer's yeast, pumpkin seeds and sunflower seeds, raisins and dried prunes, clams, nuts, tofu, kale, wheat germ, and bran.**

Selenium

This mineral is necessary for the immune system to operate properly. Some studies have shown that supplementing elderly men and women with selenium-enriched brewer's yeast increased immune function. **Sources of selenium include: whole grains, Brazil nuts, apple cider vinegar, shellfish, red swiss chard, milk, turnips, and garlic.**

Zinc

Low levels of zinc can reduce the ability to taste, slow wound healing, and decrease the ability of the body to defend itself. Several studies have indicated that elderly people may have an inadequate dietary intake of zinc or impaired absorption of zinc. Since zinc requires an acid environment to be absorbed, seniors with low stomach acid may be at risk for deficiency. **Sources of zinc include: ginger root, nuts, whole grains, chicken, shellfish, split peas, lima beans, soy lecithin, sardines, anchovies, haddock, turnips, potatoes, and garlic.**

Water

Water is necessary to prevent indigestion, constipation, and to keep the kidneys functioning properly. Unfortunately, many seniors lose their sense of thirst, making dehydration a serious problem. Excessive water loss can also be the result of diuretic therapy, diarrhea, vomiting, drinking alcohol, or drinking excessive amounts of coffee or tea. Dehydration can be recognized by dry lips, a sunken look to the eyes, elevated temperature, scant urination, constipation, nausea, and confusion. To keep the body hydrated drink at least eight glasses of fluid each day. **Good sources include: vegetable juices, diluted fruit juices, plain water, herbal teas, soymilk, and cow's milk.**

DIETARY GUIDELINES
FOR SUCCESSFUL AGING

1. Eat four or five smaller meals a day rather than three large ones. This will help to prevent indigestion. Otherwise continue to follow the disease prevention diet in Chapter 14.

2. Drink no more than two or three cups of coffee or tea a day. The caffeine in these beverages can cause dehydration and nervousness. Some studies have also linked coffee drinking with increased risk of hip fractures.

3. Dilute all fruit juices with water and decrease the amount of sweets you eat. The senior body produces less insulin and is not able to cope with large increases in blood sugar.

4. Substitute fortified soymilk for cow's milk. As some people age, they loose the ability to make lactase, the enzyme that digests lactose or milk sugar. The undigested lactose causes diarrhea, bloating, gas, and cramps. If you suspect you may have this problem, try taking a lactase supplement whenever you drink milk or eat a dairy product. Or, you can switch to soymilk that contains no lactose. Fortified soymilk is a good source of protein, calcium, and vitamin D.

5. Supplement your diet with a B-complex vitamin. Thiamin (B-1), riboflavin (B-2), and pyridoxine (B-6) have been found to lessen symptoms of depression and improve cognitive function in seniors. These vitamins are cofactors in the production of the neurotransmitters in the brain that are associated with mood and cognitive function.

6. If you take a vitamin supplement, choose one that is designed to easily break apart in a low acid stomach. Good choices include vitamins in gelatin capsules, chewable vitamins, and vitamin tablets designed to swell and burst apart in water. Bad choices include vitamins with hard coatings that require stomach acid to dissolve.

7. Drink at least eight glasses of fluid a day. This will help to prevent dehydration and constipation.

8. If chewing is painful or difficult:

- Steam vegetables and mash.
- Eat softer foods that require less chewing such as bananas, mashed potatoes and yams, macaroni and cheese, spaghetti, soups, refried beans, and quinoa (an easy-to-chew grain that is also a complete protein).
- Moisten dry food with milk or juices.
- Grind, grate, and chop raw foods as an alternative to cooking them.
- Instead of eating ground hamburger or turkey, which are often high in fat, cook lean meat or skinless poultry, chop or grind, and moisten with sauces, milk, or juices.

9. If appetite loss is a problem:

- Ask your physician or pharmacist if it could be a side effect of a drug you are taking.
- Increase foods high in thiamin and zinc. Deficiencies in these nutrients can cause appetite loss.
- Put a tablespoon of lemon juice into a glass of water and drink one half hour before mealtime. This will help to stimulate saliva, stomach acid and digestive juices.
- Try some of the meal-in-a-glass recipes in the recipe section. It is sometimes more appetizing to drink than eat.
- Drink soups fortified with vegetable juices.

10. If depression or mental fogginess is a problem:

- Ask your physician or pharmacist if it could be a side effect of a drug or combinations of drugs that you are taking. Older individuals metabolize drugs differently than younger people and overmedicating is a common problem.

- Make sure you are drinking enough fluids. A sign of dehydration is mental confusion.
- You may be taking too many over-the-counter drugs. For example, antacids can interfere with the absorption of thiamin. A deficiency of this vitamin can cause depression, insomnia, and forgetfulness.
- Take a vitamin B complex supplement each day. Thiamin, riboflavin, pyridoxine, folate, and cobalamin have all been implicated in depression and loss of cognitive abilities. Injections of cobalamin (vitamin B-12) may help. Ask your physician.

11. Drink two to three glasses of juice a day. You can make all your juices for the day at one time and store them in the refrigerator. Citrus juices and apple juice can be stored in the fridge for up to two days. Melon, cabbage, kale, broccoli, mustard greens, cauliflower, and bok choy juices will taste best when drunk within four to six hours. All other juices can be stored for up to a day.

JUICES FOR THE SENIOR YEARS

Apple: source of chromium and sorbitol (a natural laxative)
Broccoli: source of calcium and vitamin C
Cabbage: source of chromium, manganese, and vitamin C
Carrot: source of beta-carotene and trace minerals
Celery: source of potassium and other electrolytes
Collards: source of beta-carotene, calcium, zinc, and vitamin C
Ginger: source of zinc and blood thinners

Loose leaf lettuce: source of potassium, calcium, and phytosterols
Orange: source of flavonoids, vitamin C, and folacin
Tomato: source of lycopene and vitamin C
Turnips: source of potassium and vitamin C

JUICE RECIPES

Breakfast in a Glass

The B vitamins in this drink will not only wake up your body, they will also perk up your brain.

two handfuls of berries or 1 apple or 1 orange
1 ripe banana, peeled
1 heaping tablespoon selenium enriched brewer's yeast powder
4 ounces of lowfat plain yogurt, milk, or fortified soymilk

Juice fruit following your juicer's instructions. Combine juice with other ingredients in a blender and process until smooth. Serve immediately.

Lunch in a Glass

A protein, calcium, and calorie-rich drink. A good drink to offer when other food is being refused.

4 ounces of any fruit juice
3 ounces fortified soymilk
1 tablespoon protein powder
1 ripe banana, peeled

Combine ingredients in a blender and process until smooth. Serve immediately.

Evening Tonic

Drink this before going to bed to help relieve constipation.

2 apples, seeded
½ lemon, peeled
hot water

Juice ingredients. Pour juice into a cup and fill to top with hot water.

Tangerine Tea

A good substitute for coffee or tea. Full of vitamin C and folacin.

2 tangerines or oranges, peeled
¼-inch slice ginger root
hot water

Juice fruit with ginger. Pour into tea cup and fill cup to top with water. Can be prepared the night before and reheated in the morning.

Lunch in a Mug

A quick hot soup that is appealing when other foods are not.

2 tomatoes
3 ounces soymilk
½ vegetable broth cube (optional)
1 tablespoon chopped collard greens (or any other green leafy vegetable)

Juice tomato and combine ingredients in a saucepan, heat gently (being careful not to boil mixture), and pour into mug. Or combine ingredients in a mug and microwave for 30 seconds.

Potassium Cooler

A good source of potassium and the other electrolytes and beta-carotene.

½ cantaloupe
2 or 3 stalks celery

Prepare cantaloupe according to your juicer's instructions. Juice cantaloupe and celery and serve immediately.

Salad in a Glass

This drink is rich in calcium, beta-carotene, and vitamin C.

½ head loose leaf or Romaine lettuce
2 collard leaves
½ tomato
1 carrot, top removed

Juice vegetables. Serve immediately. If taste is too strong, decrease collards and increase carrots.

Simply Orange

A tasty simple juice full of folacin, vitamin C, and selenium.

4 carrots, tops removed
2 oranges, peeled

Juice ingredients and garnish with an orange slice.

CHAPTER SIXTEEN

Pregnancy and Lactation

Of all the life cycles, reproduction is the most critical and unique. At no other time will you have so much responsibility for another's welfare, since whatever you do, your unborn child does as well. If you smoke, she smokes. If you drink alcohol, she drinks alcohol. If you take drugs, she takes drugs. If you eat growth-promoting foods, she eats growth-promoting foods. If you drink juices, she drinks juices. Give your baby the most precious gift of all, good health. Good health starts with good nutrition.

CHANGES IN THE BODY DUE TO PREGNANCY

In the early weeks of pregnancy, the body begins to change physically and biochemically. These are some of the changes which affect nutrition.

Blood Volume and Composition

Blood plasma is the fluid portion of the blood. At conception, a woman averages about 2,600 ml of plasma. This increases by 1300 ml by the thirty-fourth week, an increase of 50 percent. Because of this increase in volume, the solid portions of the blood, such as the red blood cells, serum proteins and minerals, become diluted. Red blood cell production starts to increase but during the first trimester it lags behind fluid and other tissue increases. Some authorities believe that the lack of oxygen to the rapidly growing tissues is one of the causes of morning sickness. The dilution of plasma proteins results in loss of water from the blood into the tissues. This is one of the reasons for water retention during pregnancy.

Respiration

In an effort to supply more oxygen for growing tissues in the mother and fetus, more blood vessels grow in the respiratory tract as a result of stimulation by estrogen. Capillaries become distended and engorged, causing edema and congestion in the nose, larynx, trachea, and lungs. This is what causes the stuffy sensations in the nose, nosebleeds, earaches and ear stuffiness. Later in pregnancy, the growing uterus will displace the diaphragm by as much as four cm, leading to difficulty in breathing.

Kidney Function

The kidneys of the pregnant woman must not only deal with the increase in maternal wastes but those of the fetus as well. This results in an increase in filtration rate facilitated by the increase in blood volume. Normally the kidneys excrete excess water and reabsorb glucose, amino acids, and water soluble vitamins. In the overtaxed kidneys of the pregnant woman however, water is less efficiently excreted, leading to edema in the tissues, and the nutrients usually reabsorbed are lost in the urine.

Gastrointestinal Function

The pregnant woman experiences a relaxation of the smooth muscles of the body. This allows the uterus to expand. However, this muscle relaxation slows down the movement of food through the digestive tract that can result in indigestion, constipation, and hemorrhoids. Relaxation of the lower esophageal sphincter (LES) results in the splashing of stomach acid into the esophagus, causing heartburn. In addition, intestinal secretions are reduced, the absorption of nutrients is increased, and the sense of taste is changed.

NUTRIENTS NEEDED DURING PREGNANCY

The baby will grow best when the mother is able to accumulate stores of nutrients. If Mom is not well nourished, she and the baby will compete for nutrients, increasing the risk of fetal death.

Protein

Protein provides the building blocks of the placenta and the fetus. It is currently recommended that you eat sixty grams of protein a day, which is an increase of ten to sixteen grams above normal requirements. This requirement is easily met by drinking an extra two or three glasses of fortified soymilk.

Energy

A pregnant woman needs to increase her caloric intake by three hundred calories. This is usually met by eating foods to increase other nutrients.

Folacin (Folic Acid)

This B vitamin is needed for the manufacture of more blood cells for the mother and for DNA synthesis for the fetus and placental growth. Supplementation with this vitamin has been shown to decrease the incidence of neural tube defects in the fetus. **Sources of folacin include: brewer's yeast, soy flour and beans, wheat germ, beans, lentils, walnuts and filbert nuts, peanuts, and split peas.**

Pyridoxine (Vitamin B-6)

This B vitamin is needed in increased amounts for the synthesis of amino acids and niacin. Women who have taken oral contraceptives may have reduced levels of this vitamin. Some studies have shown that supplementation with seventy-five mg of pyridoxine taken in divided doses over the day reduces nausea in the first trimester of pregnancy. Ask your physician or midwife about supplementation. **Sources of pyridoxine include: brewer's yeast, sunflower seeds, wheat germ, fish, beans, nuts, bananas, and whole wheat flour.**

Ascorbic Acid (Vitamin C)

Low plasma levels of this vitamin have been associated with pre-eclampsia and premature rupture of the membranes. Pregnant women need at least 70 mg/day. This amount is easily obtained in one glass of fresh citrus juice. **Other sources of vitamin C include: guavas, sweet peppers, kale, parsley, collards, broccoli, Brussels sprouts, mustard greens, watercress, cauliflower, persimmons, red cabbage, strawberries, and papayas.**

Vitamin B-12

Low maternal B-12 levels are associated with prematurity and occur more often in smokers than nonsmokers. **Sources of B-12 include: shellfish, fish, egg yolks, lean beef. Vegans should supplement this vitamin.**

Vitamin D

This vitamin helps the fetal tissues to better utilize calcium for skeletal growth. **Sources of vitamin D include: canned sardines, salmon, fresh tuna, shrimp, sunflower seeds, eggs, mushrooms, fortified cow's milk, and fortified soymilk.**

Vitamin K

This vitamin is needed for coagulation of blood to prevent hemorrhaging after birth. **Sources of vitamin K include: turnip greens, broccoli, lettuce, cabbage, watercress, asparagus, oats, green peas, whole wheat, green beans, and eggs.**

Calcium

Calcium is needed for the fetal skeleton and for storage in the maternal skeleton for lactation. If not enough calcium is stored in the mother, the baby can leach calcium after birth, leading to maternal osteoporosis. Pregnant women need twice as much calcium as nonpregnant women. **Sources of calcium include: low-fat cow's milk, calcium fortified soymilk, collard leaves, kale, turnip greens, tofu, nonfat yogurt, goat's milk, broccoli, and romaine lettuce.**

Iron

Many women enter pregnancy with iron-deficiency anemia or reduced iron stores. Pregnant women need twice as much iron as nonpregnant women due to the increase in red blood cells. The baby must build up stores in its liver to see it through the first five to six months after birth. In order to meet these increased needs, supplementation is often recommended. Ask your physician or midwife what her recommendation is. **Sources of iron include: lean red meat, brewer's yeast, pumpkin seeds and sunflower seeds, raisins and dried prunes, clams, nuts, tofu, kale, wheat germ, and bran.**

Zinc

The amount of zinc the fetus gets comes from the mother's diet since the maternal stores in bones are not available. Malformation rates and poor pregnancy outcomes are more common in populations where zinc deficiency occurs. Zinc needs are highest early in pregnancy. An additional three to five mg of zinc is advised. This amount can be obtained by eating one cup of baked beans. **Sources of zinc include: ginger root, nuts, whole grains, chicken, shellfish, split peas, lima beans, soy lecithin, sardines, anchovies, haddock, turnips, potatoes, and garlic.**

Sodium

The metabolism of sodium is altered during pregnancy. In the past it was thought that water retention during pregnancy was due to too much sodium and women were often told to restrict the amount of salt they used. Today, mild water retention is considered normal. Women with mild edema produce fewer premature babies and babies that weigh more. Salt restriction, on the other hand, has been found to cause complications. The pregnant woman should salt her food to taste. The total amount of sodium consumed should not fall below two to three grams.

NUTRIENTS NEEDED FOR LACTATION

What the infant does not store before birth must be obtained from breastmilk after birth, making the diet of the lactating woman just as important as the diet of the pregnant woman. In general, the breastfeeding mother should follow the same nutritional advice as the pregnant women with these modifications.

Energy

More energy is needed by the lactating mother than by the pregnant women. Milk production requires about 500 extra calories a day. For the first three months about 150 to 300 of those calories can come from the fat pads laid down during pregnancy for lactation, and after that the mother must obtain all of the extra energy from foods.

Calcium

Calcium needs remain the same as during pregnancy. However, the calcium content of breastmilk is not related to the calcium content of the mother's diet. If the mother is not consuming enough calcium, it will be leached from her skeleton, causing osteoporosis over time.

Protein

Lactation requires slightly more protein than pregnancy, an additional fifteen grams per day during the first six months and twelve grams per day during the second six months.

Fluids

The nursing mother should drink three to four quarts of water a day. The amount of milk produced will be reduced if not enough fluids are consumed.

Other Nutrients

The amount of some nutrients in breastmilk is related to the amount the mother herself eats. This includes: zinc, selenium, vitamin D, vitamin A, beta-carotene, and vitamins B-6, B-12, folacin, and vitamin C. However, the amount of cholesterol in the mother's milk is not influenced by the mother's diet. If the mother does not get water soluble nutrients in sufficient quantities, the amount of milk produced will decrease. Vitamins that must be consumed in larger quantities during pregnancy are: vitamin A (200 micrograms more), vitamin E (1 microgram more), vitamin C (20 mg more), riboflavin (0.2 mg more), nicotinic acid (3 mg more), thiamin (0.1 mg), and zinc (5 mg).

DIETARY RECOMMENDATIONS
FOR PREGNANCY AND LACTATION

1. Never take any pill without the approval of your physician or midwife. This includes prescription drugs, over-the-counter medicines, herbal preparations, and food supplements.

2. Do not drink alcohol when you are pregnant or when you are breastfeeding. Besides being dangerous for the baby, one study has shown that babies nurse for less time if their mothers drink alcohol during pregnancy or while breast-feeding. Mothers who ate garlic had the longest nursing babies.

3. Limit the amount of caffeine-containing beverages that you consume to no more than two a day. Caffeine is believed to decrease blood flow to the uterus and placenta. It has been associated with an increased risk of birth defects and pregnancy complications. During lactation, caffeine is excreted into the milk and may cause irritability and poor sleeping patterns in your baby.

4. Eat a diet high in fiber. Eat at least five servings of raw fruits and vegetables each day. All cereal and grain products should be whole grains. This will not only increase fiber intake but will provide you with a number of trace minerals that your baby needs. A high-fiber diet will help to minimize constipation that results from lack of gastric motility.

5. Drink eight to ten glasses of water a day during pregnancy and twelve to sixteen glasses a day (three to four quarts) during lactation. During pregnancy this will help to relieve constipation. During lactation it is necessary to produce milk.

6. Salt your food to taste. Do not restrict the amount of salt you eat. The increase in plasma volume increases the body's need for sodium.

7. Drink at least three to four glasses of low-fat milk or fortified soymilk each day. These milks are excellent sources of protein, calcium, and vitamin D. Soymilk has the added benefit of containing cholesterol lowering factors as well as anticancer agents.

8. If you or the baby's father has a family history of allergies, avoid cow's milk and any other foods that cause allergic symptoms. Substitute calcium and vitamin D fortified soymilk.

9. Make sure your diet is rich in iron. The iron found in red meat is better absorbed than the iron found in plant foods. However the iron in plant foods will be better absorbed when it is eaten with a vitamin C–containing food.

10. Add a generous amount of calcium-containing foods to your daily diet. This is needed for the growing fetus and to supply calcium to the breastmilk after birth.

11. If you suffer from nausea:

- Keep the air in your bedroom fresh. Household odors can upset your stomach.
- Put some dry cereal or toast by your bed before you go to bed and eat this before getting out of bed the next morning.
- Get up slowly and eat some more of the dry cereal before cooking breakfast.
- Eat several small meals each day and avoid over-filling your stomach.
- Avoid foods that may give you gas while you are nauseated. This may include: broccoli, cabbage,

Brussels sprouts, collards, turnips, cucumbers, and onions.
- Avoid fats and fried foods. These tend to upset the stomach.
- During the day, try sipping a juice that contains ginger or ask your physician or midwife about taking ginger capsules. Ginger will alleviate nausea in some individuals.

12. If you have heartburn:

- Avoid foods and flavorings that relax the muscle at the entrance to the stomach. In the early stages of pregnancy, heartburn is caused by stomach acid splashing into the esophagus from the stomach. Foods that relax the muscle are: coffee, chocolate, caffeine-containing beverages, peppermint and spearmint oil, and ginger.
- Eat small frequent meals to avoid overfilling your stomach. This is particularly important in the later stages of pregnancy when heartburn is caused by crowding of the stomach by the growing uterus.
- Avoid lying down or bending over immediately after eating.

JUICES FOR PREGNANT AND LACTATING WOMEN

Apple: source of sorbitol (a natural laxative)
Broccoli: source of calcium, magnesium, beta-carotene, vitamin C, and folacin
Bok choy: source of iron, calcium, magnesium, beta-carotene, and vitamin C
Collards: source of calcium, zinc, manganese, and vitamin C
Citrus: source of vitamin C and folacin

Kale: source of iron, calcium, and vitamin C

Leeks: source of iron, calcium, magnesium, and folacin

Lettuce, Romaine: source of calcium, potassium, iron, vitamin C, and folacin

Lettuce, looseleaf: source of calcium, iron, and vitamin C

Mustard greens: source of iron, calcium, vitamin C, and beta-carotene

Pineapple: source of potassium, manganese, and bromelain (an enzyme that promotes digestion)

Turnip greens: source of beta-carotene, calcium, vitamin C, and folacin

JUICE RECIPES

Iron Special

The vitamin C in this drink increases the absorption of iron.

½ head loose leaf lettuce
1 sweet pepper
2 kale leaves

Juice vegetables and serve immediately.

Folate Tonic

Rich in folacin and calcium.

¼ head Romaine lettuce
2 turnip greens
2 carrots, tops removed

Juice vegetables. Serve immediately.

Calcium Tonic

Rich in calcium and magnesium that the developing baby needs for bone growth.

1 cup collard leaves
1 cup bok choy
6 carrots, tops removed

Juice ingredients. Serve immediately.

Super Sipper

Sip this between meals to help relieve nausea.

1 tangerine, peeled
1-inch-round slice pineapple
½ slice ginger root
sparkling water

Prepare pineapple according to your juicer's directions. Juice ingredients, pour over ice, and dilute with sparkling water.

Red Iron Special

High in iron and vitamin C.

1 leek
3 to 4 tomatoes

Juice ingredients and serve immediately.

Sweet Collard Cooler

A sweet way to get the calcium and iron in collard greens.

5 collard leaves
5 carrots, tops removed

Juice vegetables and serve immediately.

Citrus Chocolate Cooler

2 oranges, peeled
1 wedge lime, peeled
4 ounces cocoa flavored calcium-fortified soymilk

Juice fruit. Mix juice with soymilk and pour into glass. Garnish with an orange slice.

Lettuce Bowl

A calcium- and iron-rich salad you can drink.

4 cups mixture of Romaine and loose leaf lettuce
½ leek
1 tomato

Juice ingredients and serve immediately.

PART
—— IV ——
Glossary of Fruits and Vegetables

Each listing is followed by the nutrient content of the plant, the anutrient compounds, and the diseases and conditions it is recommended to prevent.

FRUITS

Apple (Malus sylvestris)

Nutrients: Soluble fiber (pectin), chromium, sorbitol (a natural laxative).
Anutrients: Polyphenols (antibacterial agents), glutathione (an antioxidant and anticarcinogen).
Recommended for: the prevention of constipation, high cholesterol, and noninsulin-dependent diabetes.

Apricot (Prunus armeniaca)

Nutrients: beta-carotene, potassium, and iron.
Anutrients: carotenoids (antioxidant compounds).
Recommended for: the prevention of cancer, high blood pressure, and stroke.

Blackberry (Rubuss spp.)

Nutrients: manganese, potassium.
Anutrients: saponins (compounds that may reduce plasma cholesterol levels).

Recommended for: prevention of infections, high cholesterol, and high blood pressure.

Blueberry (Vaccinium spp.)

Nutrients: vitamin C and potassium.
Anutrients: anthocyanins (a reddish-blue pigment), an unknown factor that prevents bacterial adherence to bladder wall.
Recommended for: the prevention of infections (bladder), heart disease, and stroke.

Cantaloupe (Cucumis melo)

Nutrients: beta-carotene, vitamin C, potassium.
Anutrients: carotenoids (yellow and red pigments that act as antioxidants), adenosine (a purine nucleoside which prevents blood clotting), glutathione (an antioxidant and anticarcinogen).
Recommended for: the prevention of infections, cancer, heart disease, and stroke.

Carambola or Starfruit (Averrhoa carambola)

Nutrients: vitamin C and potassium.
Recommended for: the prevention of infections, cancer, heart disease, and stroke.

Cherry (Prunus avium)

Nutrients: potassium.
Anutrients: anthocyanins (red pigments).
Recommended for: the prevention of infections, heart disease, high blood pressure, stroke, and gout.

Cranberry (Vaccinium macrocarpon)

Nutrients: vitamin C.
Anutrients: proanthocyanidins ("colorless" pigments) and an unknown factor that prevents the adherence of bacteria to the bladder wall.
Recommended for: prevention of infections (bladder)

Grapefruit (Citrus paradisi)

Nutrients: soluble fiber (pectin), vitamin C, folacin, potassium, and biotin.
Anutrients: flavonoids (yellow-colored pigments that have anti-inflammatory, enzyme modulatory, and antioxidant properties.), limonene (a citrus oil that blocks cancer).
Recommended for: the prevention of high cholesterol, infections, heart disease, high blood pressure, and stroke.

Grape (Vitis spp.)

Nutrients: manganese and potassium.
Anutrients: caffeic acid (a blocking agent that may prevent cancer), tannins (may be antiviral).
Recommended for: the prevention of infections, heart disease, cancer, and stroke.

Guava (Psidium guajava)

Nutrients: vitamin C and potassium.
Recommended for: the prevention of infections, heart disease, cancer, and stroke.

Honeydew Melon (Cucumis melo)

Nutrients: vitamin C and potassium.

Recommended for: prevention of cancer, heart disease, high blood pressure, and stroke.

Kiwi Fruit (Actinidia chinensis)

Nutrients: vitamin C, potassium, and magnesium.
Recommended for: prevention of cancer, heart disease, stroke, high blood pressure, infections.

Lemon (Citrus limon)

Nutrients: vitamin C and potassium.
Anutrients: Flavonoids (yellow pigments that have anti-inflammatory, enzyme inhibitory, and anti-oxidant properties), quercitin (a flavonoid that inhibits the carcinogenic effects of cooked meat and fish), monoterpenes (inhibits carcinogen activation).
Recommended for: prevention of infections, cancer, heart disease, stroke, and high blood pressure.

Lime (Citrus aurantiifolia)

Nutrients: vitamin C and potassium.
Anutrients: Flavonoids (yellow pigments that have anti-inflammatory, enzyme inhibitory, and antioxidant properties), quercitin (a flavonoid that inhibits the carcinogenic effects of cooked meat and fish), monoterpenes (inhibits carcinogen activation).
Recommended for: prevention of infections, cancer, heart disease, stroke, and high blood pressure.

Mango (Mangifera indica)

Nutrients: vitamin C, vitamin E, beta-carotene, potassium.
Anutrients: carotenoids (antioxidant pigments).

Recommended for: prevention of infections, cancer, heart disease, stroke, and high blood pressure.

Nectarine (Prunus persica var. nectarina)

Nutrients: beta carotene, potassium.
Recommended for: prevention of infections, heart disease, cancer.

Orange (Citrus sinensis)

Nutrients: vitamin C, potassium, and folacin.
Anutrients: flavonoids (yellow pigments that have anti-inflammatory, enzyme inhibitory, and antioxidant properties), quercitin (a flavonoid that inhibits the carcinogenic effects of cooked meat and fish), glutathione (an antioxidant and anticarcinogen), monoterpenes (inhibits carcinogen activation).
Recommended for: the prevention of infections, cancer, heart disease, stroke, high blood pressure.

Papaya (Carica papaya)

Nutrients: beta-carotene, vitamin C, and potassium.
Anutrients: carotenoids (antioxidant pigments), papain (an enzyme that may have anti-inflammatory properties).
Recommended for: the prevention of cancer, heart disease, high blood pressure, stroke, infections.

Peach (Prunus persica)

Nutrients: beta carotenes, potassium
Anutrients: phytosterols (plant estrogens), glutathione (an antioxidant and anticarcinogen).
Recommended for: the prevention of infections, can-

cer, heart disease, stroke, high blood pressure, and menopausal symptoms.

Pear (Pyrus communis)

Nutrients: potassium
Anutrients: phytosterols (plant estrogens), glutathione (an antioxidant and anticarcinogen).
Recommended for: the prevention of high blood pressure, stroke, and menopausal symptoms.

Pineapple (Ananas comosus)

Nutrients: potassium, manganese.
Anutrients: phytosterols, bromelain (an enzyme that may reduce inflammation, promote protein digestion, reduce platelet aggregation, improve angina pain, and reduce high blood pressure).
Recommended for: the prevention of high blood pressure, stroke, and menopausal symptoms.

Plum (Prunus spp.)

Nutrients: potassium
Anutrients: phytosterols, polyphenols (compounds that may have an antiviral activity).
Recommended for: the prevention of high blood pressure, stroke, menopausal symptoms.

Strawberry (Fragaria X ananassa)

Nutrients: vitamin C, potassium, manganese, and biotin.
Anutrients: phytosterols, polyphenols (compounds that may have antiviral activity), glutathione (an antioxidant and anticarcinogen).

Recommended for: the prevention of infections, cancer, heart disease, stroke, high blood pressure, menopausal symptoms.

Tangerine (Cirus reticulata)

Nutrients: vitamin C, potassium, folacin.
Anutrients: flavonoids (antioxidant pigments).
Recommended for: the prevention of infections, heart disease, cancer, stroke, high blood pressure.

Watermelon (Citrullus lanatus)

Nutrients: potassium, biotin.
Recommended for: high blood pressure and stroke.

VEGETABLES

Asparagus (Asparagus officinalis)

Nutrients: beta-carotene, vitamin C, vitamin E, and folacin.
Anutrients: phytosterols (plant estrogens), saponins (compounds that may reduce plasma cholesterol levels), glutathione (an antioxidant and anticarcinogen).
Recommended for: the prevention of infections, cancer, heart disease, stroke, high blood pressure, menopausal symptoms.

Beet (Beta vulgaris)

Nutrients: potassium and folacin.
Anutrients: phytosterols (plant estrogens) and glutathione (an antioxidant and anticancer compound).

Recommended for: the prevention of high blood pressure, stroke.

Beet Greens (Beta vulgaris)

Nutrients: magnesium, beta-carotene, vitamin C, vitamin E.
Anutrients: carotenoids (antioxidant pigments).
Recommended for: the prevention of cancer, heart disease, stroke.

Bell Peppers (Capsicum annuum)

Nutrients: beta-carotene, potassium, iron, zinc, vitamin C.
Anutrients: phytosterols and carotenes.
Recommended for: the prevention of infections, heart disease, stroke, high blood pressure, and menopausal symptoms.

Bok Choy (Brassica rapa)

Nutrients: Calcium, magnesium, potassium, beta-carotene, and vitamin C.
Anutrients: aromatic isothiocyanates, glucobrassicin, and indoles (cancer-blocking agents).
Recommended for: pregnant and lactating women, children, and for the prevention of infections, cancer, heart disease, high blood pressure, stroke, and osteoporosis.

Broccoli (Brassica oleracea, Botrytis Group)

Nutrients: calcium, beta-carotene, vitamin C, magnesium, and folacin.
Anutrients: carotenoids (antioxidant pigments), phytosterols (plant estrogens), aromatic isothio-

cyanates, glucobrassicin, and indoles (cancer-blocking agents), and glutathione (an antioxidant and anticarcinogen).

Recommended for: pregnant and lactating women and children and for the prevention of infections, cancer, heart disease, stroke, menopausal symptoms, and osteoporosis.

Brusells Sprouts (Brassica oleracea, Gemmifera Group)

Nutrients: calcium, magnesium, potassium, manganese, iron, beta-carotene, folacin, and vitamin C.

Anutrients: phytosterols (plant estrogens), aromatic isothiocyanates, glucobrassicin, and indoles (cancer-blocking agents).

Recommended for: pregnant and lactating women and children and for the prevention of cancer, heart disease, stroke, high blood pressure, infections, menopausal symptoms, and osteoporosis.

Cabbage (Brassica oleracea, Capitata Group)

Nutrients: potassium, vitamin C, vitamin E, and folacin.

Anutrients: phytosterols (plant estrogens), aromatic isothiocyanates (cancer-blocking and suppressing agents), glucobrassicin, and indoles (cancer-blocking agents).

Recommended for: the prevention of cancer, heart disease, stroke, osteoporosis, menopausal symptoms.

Carrots (Daucus carota)

Nutrients: beta-carotene, potassium, and soluble fiber (pectin).

Anutrients: carotenes, glutathione (an antioxidant and

anticarcinogen), phthalides (compounds that modulate arachidonic acid and prostaglandin synthesis), and phytosterols (plant estrogens).
Recommended for: the prevention of cancer, heart disease, stroke, and infections.

Cauliflower (Brassica oleracea, Botrytis Group)

Nutrients: vitamin C and potassium.
Anutrients: phytosterols, aromatic isothiocyanates (cancer-blocking and suppressing agents), glucobrassicin, indoles (cancer-blocking agents), and glutathione (an antioxidant and anticarcinogen).
Recommended for: the prevention of cancer, heart disease, stroke, and menopausal symptoms.

Celery (Apium graveolens)

Nutrients: potassium.
Anutrients: phytosterols (plant estrogens) and phthalides (compounds that modulate arachidonic acid and prostaglandin synthesis).
Recommended for: the prevention of high blood pressure, cancer, stroke, and menopausal symptoms.

Chard, Swiss (Beta vulgaris, cicla group)

Nutrients: beta-carotene, vitamin C, iron, and potassium.
Anutrients: carotenoids (pigments that act as antioxidants).
Recommended for: the prevention of infections, heart disease, stroke, and high blood pressure.

Collards (Brassica oleracea, Acephala Group)

Nutrients: beta-carotene, calcium, potassium, zinc, manganese, and vitamin C.

Anutrients: carotenoids, indoles (cancer-blocking agents), and aromatic isothiocyanates (cancer-blocking and suppressing agents).

Recommended for: children, pregnant women, and lactating women and for the prevention of infections, cancer, heart disease, stroke, high blood pressure, osteoporosis.

Cucumber (Cucumis sativus)

Nutrients: potassium.

Anutrients: phytosterols.

Recommended for: the prevention of high blood pressure, stroke, and menopausal symptoms.

Garlic (Allium sativum)

Nutrients: zinc.

Anutrients: saponins (compounds that may reduce plasma cholesterol levels), ajoene (prevents blood clots), allicin (a natural antibiotic agent), and other organosulfur compounds (cancer-blocking and suppressive agents).

Recommended for: pregnant and lactating women and for the prevention of high cholesterol, heart disease, stroke, high blood pressure, cancer, and infections.

Ginger Root

Nutrients: zinc.

Anutrients: gingerol (prevents blood cell clumping) and other unknown compounds.

Recommended for: prevention of heart disease and stroke, nausea of pregnancy, and motion sickness.

Kale (Brassica oleracea, Acephala Group)

Nutrients: calcium, iron, potassium, manganese, magnesium, beta-carotene, and vitamin C.
Anutrients: carotenoids (pigments that act as antioxidants), aromatic isothiocyanates (cancer-blocking and suppressing agents), and indoles (cancer-blocking agents).
Recommended for: children, pregnant women, and lactating women, and for the prevention of infections, cancer, heart disease, stroke, high blood pressure, and osteoporosis.

Leeks (Allium ampeloprasum)

Nutrients: iron, potassium, magnesium, and folacin.
Anutrients: saponins (compounds that may reduce plasma cholesterol levels), and organosulfur compounds (cancer-blocking agents).
Recommended for: the prevention of infections, cancer, heart disease, stroke, high blood pressure, and high cholesterol levels.

Lettuce, Romaine (Lactuca sativa)

Nutrients: iron, potassium, beta-carotene, vitamin C, and folacin.
Anutrients: carotenoids.
Recommended for: the prevention of infections, cancer, heart disease, stroke, and high blood pressure.

Lettuce, loose leaf (Lactuca sativa)

Nutrients: calcium, iron, potassium, vitamin C, and beta-carotene.
Anutrients: phytosterols (plant estrogens) and carotenoids (antioxidant pigments).
Recommended for: children, pregnant women, and lactating women, and for the prevention of infections, cancer, heart disease, stroke, menopausal problems, and high blood pressure.

Mustard Greens (Brassica juncea)

Nutrients: calcium, iron, beta-carotene, vitamin C, vitamin E, and magnesium.
Anutrients: carotenoids (act as antioxidants) and indoles (cancer-blocking agents).
Recommended for: the prevention of infections, cancer, heart disease, stroke, high blood pressure, and osteoporosis.

Onions (Allium cepa)

Nutrients: potassium.
Anutrients: phytosterols, organosulfur compounds (cancer-blocking agents), diphenylamine (an agent that lowers blood sugar in animals), prostaglandin A1 (may lower blood pressure), a natural antibiotic compound, ajoene (prevents blood clots).
Recommended for: the prevention of infections, cancer, heart disease, stroke, high blood pressure, noninsulin-dependent diabetes, menopausal symptoms.

Parsley (Petroselinum crispum)

Nutrients: iron, potassium, folacin, and beta-carotene.

Anutrients: phthalides (compounds which modulate arachidonic acid and prostaglandin synthesis) and carotenoids (pigments with antioxidant abilities).
Recommended for: the prevention of infections, cancer, heart disease, and stroke.

Radish (Raphanus sativus)

Nutrients: potassium.
Anutrients: phytosterols and benzyl isothiocyanate (cancer-blocking agent).
Recommended for: the prevention of cancer, high blood pressure, stroke, and menopausal symptoms.

Spinach (Spinacia oleracea)

Nutrients: magnesium, potassium, manganese, beta-carotene, vitamin C, vitamin E, and folacin.
Anutrients: carotenoids (pigments that act as antioxidants), saponins (compounds that may reduce plasma cholesterol levels), and glutathione (an antioxidant and anticarcinogen).
Recommended for: the prevention of infections, heart disease, cancer, stroke, and high blood pressure.

Tomato (Lycopersicon esculentum)

Nutrients: beta-carotene, potassium, and vitamin C.
Anutrients: lycopene (a carotenoid with powerful antioxidant properties), phytosterols, and glutathione (an antioxidant and anticarcinogen).
Recommended for: the prevention of infections, cancer, heart disease, stroke, high blood pressure, and menopausal symptoms.

Turnip (Brassica rapa, Papifera group)

Nutrients: potassium and vitamin C.
Anutrients: phytosterols and benzyl isothiocyanate (cancer-blocking agent).
Recommended for: the prevention of cancer, high blood pressure, stroke, and menopausal symptoms.

Turnip Greens (Brassica rapa, Papifera group)

Nutrients: beta-carotene, calcium, iron, and potassium, manganese, vitamin C, folacin, pyridoxine, and vitamin E.
Anutrients: carotenoids (pigments with antioxidant properties) and phytosterols.
Recommended for: the prevention of infections, cancer, heart disease, stroke, high blood pressure, osteoporosis, menopausal symptoms.

REFERENCES

Aging

Schneider, E. L., and Brody, J. A., Aging, natural death and the compression of morbidity: another view. *New England Journal of Medicine,* 309:854–856, 1983.

Warner, H. R. (ed.), et al., *Modern Biological Theories of Aging.* New York: Raven Press, 1987.

Coronary Heart Disease

McNamara, D., Coronary Heart Disease. In: *Present Knowledge in Nutrition,* pp. 349–361. Washington, D.C.: International Life Sciences Institute–Nutrition Foundation, 1990.

National Research Council (U.S.), Committee on Diet and Health, *Diet and health: implications for reducing chronic disease risk.* Washington, D.C.: National Academy Press, 1991.

Simon, J. A., Vitamin C and cardiovascular disease: a review. *Journal of the American College of Nutrition,* 11:107–125, 1992.

Cancer

Beyers, T., LaChance, R. A., and Pierson, H. E., New directions: The diet-cancer link. *Patient Care,* 24:34–48, Nov. 30, 1990.

Jones, D. P., Coates, R. L., Fagg, E. W., et al., Glutathione in foods listed in the National Cancer Institute's Health Habits and History Food Frequency Questionnaire. *Nutrition and Cancer,* 17:57–73, 1992.

Messina, M., and Barnes, S., The role of soy products in reducing risk of cancer. *Journal of the National Cancer Institute,* 83:541–546, 1991.

Wattenberg, L. W., Inhibition of carcinogenesis by minor anutrient constituents of the diet. *Proceedings of the Nutrition Society,* 49:173–183, 1990.

Weisburger, J. H., Nutritional approach to cancer prevention with emphasis on vitamins, antioxidants, and carotenoids. *American Journal of Clinical Nutrition,* 53:2268–2378, 1991.

Hypertension

Howe, P., Rogers, P., and Lungershausen, Y., Blood pressure reduction by fish oil in adults in adult rats with established hypertension—dependence on sodium intake. *Prost Leuko Essent Fatty Acids,* 44:113–117, 1991.

Lau, B. H., Anticoagulant and lipid regulating effects of garlic. *New Protective Roles for Selective Nutrients,* pp. 295–325.

Touyz, R., Magnesium supplementation as an adjuvant to synthetic calcium channel antagonists in the treatment of hypertension. *Medical Hypothesis*, 36: 140–141, 1991.

Stroke

National Research Council (U.S.), Committee on Diet and Health. *Diet and health: implications for reducing chronic disease risk.* Washington, D.C.: National Academy Press, 1991.

Diabetes

Hollenbeck, C. B., and Coulston, A. M., Diabetes mellitius. In: *Present Knowledge in Nutrition*, pp. 349–361. Washington, D. C.: International Life Sciences Institute–Nutrition Foundation.

Khan, A., Bryden, N., Poland, M., et al., Insulin potentiating factor and chromium content of selected foods and spices. *Biological Trace Elements Research*, 24:183–188, 1990.

Itoh, R., J. Echizen, H., et al., The interrelation of urinary calcium and sodium intake in healthy elderly Japanese. *International Journal of Vitamin and Nutrition Research*, 61:159–165, 1991.

Osteoporosis

Dawson-Hughes, B., Calcium supplementation and bone loss: a review of controlled clinical trials. *American Journal of Clinical Nutrition.* 54:2748–2808, 1991.

Sowers, M., Osteoporosis and osteomalacia. In: *Present Knowledge in Nutrition*, pp. 349–361. Washington, D.C.: International Life Sciences Institute–Nutrition Foundation.

Tobacco-Related Diseases

Preston, A. M., Cigarette smoking—nutritional implications. *Progress in Food and Nutrition Science,* Vol. 15, pp. 183–217, 1991.

Immune functioning

Jacob, R., Kelly, D., Pianalto, F., et al., Immunocompetence and oxidant defense during ascorbate depletion of healthy men. *American Journal of Clinical Nutrition,* 54:13028–13098, 1991.

Infants and Children

Pipes, P. L., *Nutrition in Infancy and Childhood.* St. Louis, Missouri: Times Mirror/Mosby College Publishing, 1989.

Lozoff, B., and Wolf, A., Long-term developmental outcome of infants with iron deficiency. *New England Journal of Medicine,* 325:687–694, 1991.

Adolescents and Young Adults

Dawson, E., Harris, W., and Powell, L., Effects of vitamin C supplementation of sperm quailty of heavy smokers, *FASEBJ,* 5(4):A915, 1991.

Mahan, L. K., and Rees, J. M., *Nutrition in Adolescence.* St. Louis, Missouri: Times Mirror/Mosby College Publishing.

Senior Adults

Bell, I., Edman, J., Morrow, E., et al., B-complex vitamin patterns in geriatric and young adult inpatients with major depression. *Journal of the American Geriatric Society,* 39:252–257, 1991.

Katahn, M., Nutrition and older persons: A clinical perspective. *The Nutrition Report,* Volume 8, No 12, 1991.

Mobarhan, S., Hupert, J., and Friedman, H., Effects of aging on beta-carotene and vitamin A status. *Age,* 14:13–16, 1991.

Penn, N., Purkins, L., Kelleher, J., et al., The effect of dietary supplementation with vitamins A, C, and E on cell-mediated immune function in elderly long-stay patients: A randomized controlled trial. *Age,* 20:169–174, 1991.

Pregnancy and Lactation

MRC Vitamin Research Group, Prevention of neural tube defects: results of the Medical Research Council Vitamin Study. Lancet 338:131–137, 1991.

Nakamoto, T., Gottschalk, S., Yazdani, M., et al., Combined effects of caffeine and zinc in the maternal diet on fetal brains. *FASEBJ,* 5:A1319, 1991.

Sahakian, V., Rouse, D., Dipes, S., et al., Vitamin B-6 is effective therapy for nausea and vomiting of pregnancy: a randomized double-blind placebo-controlled study. *Obstet Gynecol,* 78:33–36, 1991.

Worthington-Roberts, B., and Williams, S. R., *Nutrition in Pregnancy and Lactation,* St. Louis, Missouri: Times Mirror/Mosby College Publishing, 1980.